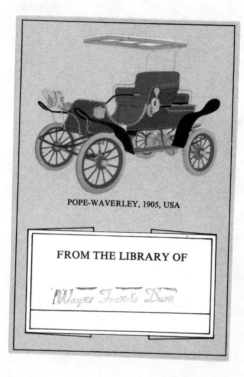

POPE-WAVERLEY, 1905, USA

Current
Medical
Abbreviations

The
Charles Press
Handbook of
Current Medical
Abbreviations

The Charles Press Publishers, Inc.

Bowie, Maryland

The Charles Press Handbook of Current Medical Abbreviations

Library of Congress Cataloging in Publication Data
Main entry under title:

The Charles Press handbook of current medical abbreviations.

1. Medicine—Abbreviations. I. Charles Press Publishers. [DNLM: 1. Medicine—Abbreviations. W13 C476]
R121.C438   610'.1'48   76-40101
ISBN 0-913486-80-9

Prentice-Hall International, Inc., London

Prentice-Hall of Australia, Pty., Ltd., Sydney

Prentice-Hall of India Private Limited, New Delhi

Prentice-Hall of Japan, Inc., Tokyo

Prentice-Hall of Southeast Asia Pte. Ltd., Singapore

Whitehall Books Limited, Wellington, New Zealand

Printed in the United States of America

78 79 80 81 82   10 9 8 7 6 5 4 3 2

Preface

"What in the world does this mean? It says the patient is scheduled for a CABG."

"I don't know. Look it up in the medical dictionary."

"I did. It isn't there."

"Ask the nursing supervisor, she may know."

"She had no idea."

"Try the chemistry lab, maybe it's a special test."

"They never heard of it."

"Dr. Smith is here, ask him."

"He just shook his head."

"Well, it must be a new abbreviation for something."

"But for what?"

This dialogue will be very familiar to hospital personnel and to all others who must interpret medical abbreviations. New abbreviations appear so rapidly that it is difficult to stay abreast with them. This problem is not likely to improve; in fact, it will probably get worse. Each new operation, disease, test, procedure, technique, or other innovation in medicine brings with it a new abbreviation, and, with medical progress being as swift as it now is, more and more abbreviations can surely be expected each year. Furthermore, medical records-keeping has become such a tedious and time consuming task that physicians have resorted to abbreviating as many words as they can—a practice that can only continue to increase.

The purpose of this handbook is to provide a listing of common medical abbreviations in *clinical* use at the present time. Because the book focuses on clinical usage, only those abbreviations that would normally be found on a patient's chart are included. Abbreviations that are no longer popular, or are obsolete, have been deliberately excluded.

To enhance the overall usefulness of the book we have added parenthetical notes to explain certain abbreviations, particularly those that have multiple meanings and those derived from Latin. Abbreviations related to physicians' orders have been qualified to indicate whether they refer to medications, procedures, x-ray studies, diet orders, intravenous therapy, operations, or laboratory tests. The laboratory tests have been further delineated in terms of which laboratory slip should be used in ordering a particular test.

We are grateful to the more than 30 consultants who helped to compile the abbreviations presented in this book. They included nurses, physicians in nearly all specialties, pharmacists, laboratory staffs, and medical record librarians in representative community and teaching hospitals. A special note of appreciation must go to Eileen Sankey, R.N. and Elizabeth Meholick who prepared the final manuscript.

The Charles Press, Publishers, Inc.
September 1976

Since we plan to revise and update this book periodically, we shall be very pleased to receive any suggestions regarding new abbreviations that should be included in the next edition. Please forward your suggestions to the Editor-in-Chief, The Charles Press Publishers, Inc., Bowie, Maryland 20715.

Current
Medical
Abbreviations

A

A	adult anterior artery assessment (in problem-oriented medical records)
a	accommodation (eye examination) ampere
A_1	aortic first heart sound
A_2	aortic second heart sound
$\bar{a}$	before (Latin: *ante*)
AA	achievement age (pediatrics) Alcoholics Anonymous ascending aorta atomic absorption (laboratory method) Australia antigen (laboratory/serology)
aa (aa)	of each (medication orders/prescriptions)
AAA	abdominal aortic aneurysm
$A\text{-a}DO_2$	alveolar-arterial oxygen difference (pulmonary function test)
AAL	anterior axillary line
AAO	amino acid oxidase
Ab	antibody
ab.	abortion
abd.	abdomen (abdominal) abduction
Abd. Hyst.	abdominal hysterectomy (operation/gynecology)

abdom.	abdomen (abdominal)
ABE	acute bacterial endocarditis
ABG	arterial blood gases (laboratory/blood gas)
ABP	arterial blood pressure
ABR	absolute bed rest
ABS	acute brain syndrome
abs.	absent absolute
abs. feb.	in the absence of fever (Latin: *absente febre*)
aby.	antibody
AC	adrenal cortex air conduction (hearing test) alternating current anterior chamber (eye examination)
A/C	anchored catheter
ac.	acid acute
a.c.	before meals (Latin: *ante cibum*) (medication orders/prescriptions)
acc.	accident according
accom.	accommodation (eye examination)
ACD	absolute cardiac dullness anterior chest diameter
Acet.	acetone
ACG	apexcardiogram (procedure/cardiology)
ac. phos.	acid phosphatase (laboratory/chemistry)

acid phos.	acid phosphatase (laboratory/chemistry)
acid p'tase.	acid phosphatase (laboratory/chemistry)
ACT	activated clotting time (laboratory/coagulation)
ACTH	adrenocorticotrophic hormone (medication order)
ACU	acute care unit
AD	right ear (Latin: *auris dextra*)
ADA diet	American Diabetic Association diet
add.	adduction
ADE	acute disseminated encephalitis
adenoca.	adenocarcinoma (cancer)
ADH	antidiuretic hormone
ADL	activities of daily living
ad lib	as desired (Latin: *ad libitum*)
adm.	admission
admin.	administer
ADP	adenosine diphosphate
ADR	adverse drug reaction (report)
ADT	adenosine triphosphate
AEG	air encephalogram (procedure/neurology)
AF	atrial fibrillation
Af	atrial flutter
AFB	acid-fast bacillus (tuberculosis) (laboratory/bacteriology)
A fib.	atrial fibrillation

AFP	alpha-feroprotein (laboratory/chemistry)
agglut.	agglutination
agit.	shake (Latin: *agita*) (medication orders/prescriptions)
AGL	acute granulocytic leukemia
AGN	acute glomerulonephritis
$AgNO_3$ sol.	silver nitrate solution (medication orders/prescriptions)
A/G ratio	albumin/globulin ratio (laboratory/chemistry)
AGS	adrenogenital syndrome
AHA	autoimmune hemolytic anemia
AHD	antihypertensive drug arteriosclerotic heart disease autoimmune hemolytic disease
AHF	antihemophilic factor (laboratory/coagulation)
AI	aortic insufficiency
AID	acute infectious disease artificial insemination–donor
AIH	artificial insemination–husband
AJ	ankle jerk
AK	above knee (operation/amputation)
alb.	albumin (laboratory/chemistry)
ALD	alcoholic liver disease
ALG	antilymphocytic globulin
alk.	alkaline

alk. phos.	alkaline phosphatase (laboratory/chemistry)
alk. p'tase.	alkaline phosphatase (laboratory/chemistry)
ALL	acute lymphocytic leukemia
ALS	amyotrophic lateral sclerosis
alt.	alternate
alv.	alveolar
AM	before noon (Latin: *ante meridianus*)
AMA	against medical advice
AMAP	as much as possible
amb.	ambulate (ambulatory)
AMI	acute myocardial infarction
AML	acute myelogenous leukemia
ammon.	ammonia
amorph.	amorphous
AMP	adenosine monophosphate ampicillin (on culture and sensitivity reports) average mean pressure
amp.	ampere ampule (medication order) amputation
amphet.	amphetamine
A–M prosthesis	Austin–Moore prosthesis
amt.	amount
ANA	antinuclear antibody (laboratory/serology)
anes.	anesthesia (anesthetic)

ANF	antinuclear factor (laboratory/serology)
angio.	angiogram (procedure/cardiovascular)
aniso.	anisocytosis (of red blood cells)
ANLL	acute nonlymphocytic leukemia
ANS	arteriolonephrosclerosis autonomic nervous system
ant.	anterior
ant. ax. line	anterior axillary line
AOB	alcohol on breath
AOD	arterial occlusive disease
aort. regurg.	aortic regurgitation
aort. sten.	aortic stenosis
AP	alkaline phosphatase (laboratory/chemistry) angina pectoris ante partum (obstetrics) anterior pituitary anteroposterior aortic pressure apical pulse appendectomy artificial pneumothorax
A-P	anterior-posterior
A & P	auscultation and percussion
$A_2 > P_2$	aortic second sound is greater than pulmonic second sound
APB	atrial premature beat
APC's	atrial premature contractions

APC tabs.	aspirin, phenacetin, and caffeine tablets (medication orders/prescriptions)
A-P D	anteroposterior diameter
APH	ante partum hemorrhage (obstetrics)
A-P & Lat.	anterior-posterior and lateral (x-ray/chest)
appl.	appliance application applied
appt.	appointment
A-P repair	anterior-posterior repair (operation/gynecology)
APTT	activated partial thromboplastin time (laboratory/coagulation)
aq.	aqueous
aq. dist.	distilled water (Latin: *aqua distillata*) (medication orders/prescriptions)
AR	aortic regurgitation apical rate
A/R	apical/radial (pulse)
ARB	any reliable brand (medication orders/prescriptions)
ARD	acute respiratory disease
ARDS	adult respiratory distress syndrome
ARF	acute renal failure acute respiratory failure acute rheumatic fever
AS	aortic stenosis arteriosclerosis left ear (Latin: *auris sinistra*)

ASA	acetylsalicylic acid (aspirin) (medication orders/prescriptions)
ASAP	as soon as possible
A-S attack	Adams-Stokes attack
ASCVD	arteriosclerotic cardiovascular disease
ASD	atrial septal defect
ASH	asymmetrical septal hypertrophy
ASHD	arteriosclerotic heart disease
ASLO titer	antistreptolysin-O titer (laboratory/serology)
ASO titer	antistreptolysin-O titer (laboratory/serology)
assn.	association
assoc.	associated
as tol	as tolerated
ASV	antisnake venom
at. fib	atrial fibrillation
ATG	antithymocyte globulin
ATN	acute tubular necrosis
ATP	adenosine triphosphate
AU	both ears (Latin: *aures unitas*)
^{198}Au	radioactive gold (nuclear medicine)
AV	aortic valve atrioventricular
-V	arteriovenous
AVF	augmented V lead, left leg (ECG)
AVL	augmented V lead, left arm (ECG)

AVN	atrioventricular node
AVR	aortic valve replacement (operation/cardiac) augmented V lead, right arm (ECG)
AVS	arteriovenous shunt
Ax.	axillary
ax.	axis
A & W	alive and well

B

B	bacillus basophil (on white blood count reports) black brother Brucella (on bacteriology reports)
b	born
BA	blood agar (culture medium) bone age brachial artery bronchial asthma
Ba.	barium
bact.	bacteria (bacterial)
Ba. E	barium enema (x-ray/colon)
BAL	British anti-lewisite (medication order)
bands	banded neutrophils (on white blood count reports)

barb.	barbiturate
baso.	basophils (on white blood count reports)
Ba. swallow	barium swallow (x-ray/esophagus)
BB	blood bank both bones (regarding fractures) breakthrough bleeding
BBA	born before arrival
BBB	bundle branch block (ECG)
BBBB	bilateral bundle branch block (ECG)
BBT	basal body temperature
B Bx.	breast biopsy
BC	birth control blood culture (laboratory/bacteriology) Blue Cross bone conduction (hearing test)
B & C	bed and chair (rest) biopsy and curettage (operation/gynecology)
BCC	basal cell carcinoma
BCE	basal cell epithelioma
BCG	bacille Calmette Guérin ballistocardiogram (procedure/cardiology)
BCN	bilateral cortical necrosis
BD	bile duct bottle drainage

BE	bacterial endocarditis
	barium enema
	(x-ray/colon)
	below elbow
	(operation/amputation)
BEI	butanol extractable iodine
	(thyroid test)
	(laboratory/chemistry)
bev	billion electron volts
	(radiation therapy)
BF	black female
	blood flow
BFP	biological false positive (test)
BFR	blood flow rate
	bone formation rate
BFR sol.	buffered Ringer's solution
	(intravenous solution)
BG	blood glucose
	(laboratory/chemistry)
	bone graft
	(operation/orthopedics)
BHS	beta-hemolytic streptococcus
BI	burn index
bib.	drink (Latin: *bibe*)
	(medication order)
b.i.d.	twice a day (Latin: *bis in die*)
bilat.	bilateral
bili.	bilirubin
	(laboratory/chemistry)
bili. D/I	bilirubin, direct and indirect
	(laboratory/chemistry)

BISp	between ischial spines (pelvic measurement)
bisp. diam.	bispinous diameter (pelvic measurement)
BJ	biceps jerk bone and joint
BJM	bones, joints, muscles
BJ protein	Bence-Jones protein (laboratory/urine)
BKA	below knee amputation (operation/orthopedics)
bkfst.	breakfast
bl.	bleeding blood blue
bl. cult.	blood culture (laboratory/bacteriology)
bl. obs.	bladder observation
BLT	blood-clot lysis time
Bl. T	blood type
bl. time	bleeding time (laboratory/coagulation)
bl. x	bleeding time (laboratory/coagulation)
BM	basal metabolism black male body mass bone marrow bowel movement
BMR	basal metabolic rate

BNDD	Bureau of Narcotics and Dangerous Drugs (physician's narcotic number)
BNO	bladder neck obstruction
BO	body odor bowel obstruction
B & O	belladonna and opium (medication orders/prescriptions)
bol.	bolus (medication orders/prescriptions)
BP	back pressure bedpan birthplace blood pressure bronchopleural bypass (operation/cardiovascular)
BPH	benign prostatic hypertrophy
BR	bathroom bed rest
Br.	bromide brown
BRB	bright red blood
BRP	bathroom privileges
br. sounds	breath sounds
BS	bedside blood sugar (laboratory/chemistry) Blue Shield bowel sounds breath sounds
B & S glands	Bartholin and Skene glands

BSA	body surface area
BSB	body surface burned
BSD	bedside drainage
BSI	bound serum iron
BSO	bilateral salpingo-oophorectomy (operation/gynecology)
BSP	bromsulphalein (laboratory/chemistry)
BT	bedtime bladder tumor bleeding time (laboratory/coagulation) body temperature brain tumor breast tumor
BTB	breakthrough bleeding
BTL	bilateral tubal ligation (operation/gynecology)
BTPD	body temperature and ambient pressure, dry (in pulmonary function test reports)
BTPS	body temperature and ambient pressure, saturated with water vapor (in pulmonary function test reports)
BTU	British thermal unit
BUN	blood urea nitrogen (laboratory/chemistry)
BV	blood vessel blood volume bronchovesicular (breath sounds)

BVH	biventricular hypertrophy (heart)
BVL	bilateral vas ligation (operation/genitourinary)
BW	birth weight body weight
Bx.	biopsy

C

C	calorie (diet order) carbohydrate (diet order) Caucasian centigrade cervical chest chloramphenicol (on culture and sensitivity reports) Clostridium closure correct Cryptococcus (on bacteriology reports) cylinder (eye examination) hundred (Latin: *centum*) (medication orders/prescriptions)
c	capacity cubic
C′	complement
C₁, C₂ . . . 	cervical vertebrae 1, 2 . . .
c̄	with (Latin: *cum*)

CA	carbonic anhydrase
	carcinoma (cancer)
	cardiac arrest
	chronological age
	cold agglutinin
	common antigen
	coronary artery
	cortisone acetate
C & A	Clinitest and Acetest (urine test/diabetes)
Ca	calcium (laboratory/chemistry)
	carcinoma (cancer)
CABG	coronary artery bypass graft (operation/open heart surgery)
CAD	coronary artery disease
CAH	chronic active hepatitis
Cal.	calorie (diet order)
cal.	caliber
C_{alb}	albumin clearance (renal function test) (laboratory/chemistry)
C_{am}	amylase clearance (laboratory/chemistry)
CAO	chronic airway obstruction
cap.	capacity
caps.	capsules (medication orders/prescriptions)
cardiol.	cardiology
Cath.	Catholic

cath.	cathartic
	catheter (catheterize)
caut.	cauterize (cauterization)
CB	carbenicillin (on culture and sensitivity reports)
C & B	chair and bed (rest)
CBC	complete blood count (laboratory/hematology)
CBD	closed bladder drainage
	common bile duct
CBF	cerebral blood flow
	coronary blood flow
CBR	complete bed rest
CBV	central blood volume
	circulating blood volume
	corrected blood volume
CC	cardiac cycle
	chief complaint
	clindamycin (on culture and sensitivity reports)
	clinical course
	cord compression
	costochondral
	creatinine clearance
	critical condition
	current complaints
cc.	cubic centimeter
CCA	common carotid artery
CCE	clubbing, cyanosis or edema
CCF	compound comminuted fracture
CCMSU	clean catch midstream urine (procedure/urine culture)

CCU	coronary care unit
CCW	counterclockwise
CD	cadaver donor (transplantations) Caesarean delivered (obstetrics) cardiac disease cardiac dullness cardiovascular disease caudal common duct conjugata diagonalis (pelvic measurement) consanguineous donor convulsive disorder cystic duct
C.D.	communicable disease
C/d	cigarettes per day
C & D	cystoscopy and dilatation (procedure/urology)
CDE	chlordiazepoxide (Librium)
CDH	congenital dislocation of the hip
CE	California encephalitis cardiac enlargement cholesterol esters (laboratory/chemistry)
CEA	carcinoembryonic antigen (laboratory/chemistry)
ceph. floc.	cephalin flocculation (laboratory/chemistry)
CF	cardiac failure cephalothin (on culture and sensitivity reports) Chiari-Frommel (syndrome) Christmas factor

	complement fixation
	contractile force
	count fingers (eye examination)
	cystic fibrosis
cf.	compare (Latin: *confero*)
CFP	chronic false positive (test)
CFT	complement fixation test (laboratory/serology)
CG	cardio-green (dye)
	chorionic gonadotropin (laboratory/chemistry)
	chronic glomerulonephritis
	colloidal gold (laboratory/serology)
CGD	chronic granulomatous disease
CGL	chronic granulocytic leukemia
CGN	chronic glomerulonephritis
CGP	chorionic growth hormone prolactin
CGS	catgut suture (surgical reports)
CGTT	cortisone glucose tolerance test (diabetes detection) (laboratory/chemistry)
CH	Community Health
	crown-heel (length of fetus)
ch.	chest
	chief
	child
CHB	complete heart block (ECG)
CHD	childhood disease
	congenital heart disease
	coronary heart disease

CHE	cholinesterase
CHF	congestive heart failure
CHO	carbohydrate (diet order)
chol.	cholesterol (laboratory/chemistry)
chol. est.	cholesterol esters (laboratory/chemistry)
chr.	chronic
CHTZ	chlorothiazide (diuretic)
CI	cardiac index cerebral infarction color index complete iridectomy (operation/ophthalmology) coronary insufficiency crystalline insulin
Ci	Curie (measurement of radioactivity)
CICU	coronary intensive care unit
CID	cytomegalic inclusion disease
CIDS	cellular immunity deficiency syndrome
circ.	circular circulation circumcision
CIS	carcinoma in situ
CK	creatine kinase (same as CPK) (laboratory/chemistry)
ck.	check (checked)
CL	chest and left arm (ECG lead) colistin (on culture and sensitivity reports)

	corpus luteum
	critical list
Cl	chloride (laboratory/chemistry)
	clavicle
	clinic
	Clostridium (on bacteriology reports)
cl.	clear
CLD	chronic liver disease
	chronic lung disease
cldy.	cloudy
CLL	chronic lymphocytic leukemia
CLT	clot-lysis time
cl. time	clotting time (laboratory/coagulation)
clysis	hypodermocylsis (procedure/fluid infusion)
CM	contrast media (dye)
	costal margin
cm.	centimeter
c.m.	tomorrow morning (Latin: *cras mane*)
cm³	cubic centimeter
CMC	carboxymethyl cellulose
CMF	cyclophosamide, methotrexate, 5-fluorouracil (cancer chemotherapy)
CMHC	Community Mental Health Center
c/min.	cycles per minute
CMO	cardiac minute output
CMV	cytomegalovirus

CN	charge nurse
C.N.	cranial nerve
CNE	chronic nervous exhaustion
CNH	community nursing home
CNS	central nervous system
CO	carbon monoxide (laboratory/chemistry) cardiac output castor oil
c/o	complains of
^{60}Co	radioactive cobalt (nuclear medicine)
CO_2	carbon dioxide
CoA	coenzyme A
coag.	coagulase (on bacteriology reports) coagulation
coag. time	coagulation time
CO_2 comb.	carbon dioxide combining power (laboratory/blood gas)
CO_2 cont.	carbon dioxide content (laboratory/blood gas)
COD	cause of death
Cod. SO_4	codeine sulfate (medication orders/prescriptions)
COHB	carboxyhemoglobin (laboratory/chemistry)
col.	colony (on culture reports) colored
COLD	chronic obstructive lung disease
commun.	communicable

comp.	compensated (heart disease)
	compensation (case)
	complaint
	complete
	complication
	composition
	compound
conc.	concentration (concentrated)
	conclusion
cond.	condition
	conduction
cont.	containing
	contents
	continue (continuously)
	contusion
conv.	convalescent
COP	capillary osmotic pressure
COPD	chronic obstructive pulmonary disease
COPE	chronic obstructive pulmonary emphysema
cort.	cortex
	cortical
	cortisone
CP	capillary pressure
	cerebral palsy
	chronic pyelonephritis
	cleft palate
	closing pressure (spinal tap)
	combining power
	coproporphyrin
	cor pulmonale
	creatine phosphate (laboratory/chemistry)

C & P	cystoscopy and panendoscopy (procedure/urology)
CPA	cerebellar pontine angle (tumor)
C_{pah}	para-aminohippurate clearance (procedure/renal function test)
CPAP	continuous positive airway pressure (respiratory therapy)
CPB	cardiopulmonary bypass
CPC	chronic passive congestion clinicopathologic conference
CPD	cephalopelvic disproportion
Cpd. E	cortisone (Compound E)
Cpd. F	hydrocortisone (Compound F)
CPE	chronic pulmonary emphysema
CPI	constitutional psychopathic inferiority
CPK	creatine phosphokinase (laboratory/chemistry)
CPN	chronic pyelonephritis
CPPB	continuous positive pressure breathing (respiratory therapy)
CPPV	continuous positive pressure ventilation (respiratory therapy)
CPR	cardiopulmonary resuscitation
C/P ratio	cholesterol-phospholipid ratio (laboratory/chemistry)
c.p.s.	cycles per second
CPT	chest physiotherapy (respiratory therapy)

CPZ	chlorpromazine (Thorazine)
CR	cardiorespiratory
	chest and right arm (ECG lead)
	clot retraction (laboratory/coagulation)
	colon resection (operation/abdominal)
	complete remission
	conditioned reflex
	crown-rump (length of fetus)
^{51}Cr	radioactive chromium (nuclear medicine)
CRA	central retinal artery
cran.	cranial (nerves)
CRBBB	complete right bundle branch block (ECG)
CRD	chronic renal disease
	chronic respiratory disease
creat.	creatine (laboratory/chemistry)
	creatinine (laboratory/chemistry)
CRF	chronic renal failure
crit.	hematocrit (laboratory/hematology)
CRP	C-reactive protein
CRT	cardiac resuscitation team
crt.	hematocrit (laboratory/hematology)
CRV	central retinal vein
crys.	crystalline (crystallized)

CS	Central Service (Central Supply)
	cerebrospinal (fluid)
	concentrated strength (drugs)
	conscious
	coronary sinus
	corticosteroid
cs.	case (cases)
	conscious (consciousness)
C & S	conjunctiva and sclera (eye examination)
	culture and sensitivity (laboratory/bacteriology)
C. section	Caesarean section (operation/obstetrics)
CSF	cerebrospinal fluid
CSH	chronic subdural hematoma
CSHEP	constriction, sclerosis, hemorrhage, exudate, papilledema (eye examination)
CSM	carotid sinus massage (cardiology)
	cerebrospinal meningitis
CSR	Central Supply Room
	Cheyne-Stokes respiration
	corrected sedimentation rate (laboratory/hematology)
CSS	carotid sinus stimulation
CST	convulsive shock therapy (procedure/psychiatry)
CT	carotid tracing
	carpal tunnel (syndrome)
	cerebral thrombosis
	chlorothiazide (diuretic)
	circulation time (procedure/cardiology)

	clotting time (laboratory/coagulation)
	coagulation time (laboratory/coagulation)
	coated tablet
	computer-assisted tomagraphy (procedure/x-ray)
	connective tissue
	Coomb's test (laboratory/blood bank)
	coronary thrombosis
ct.	count
cta.	catamenia (menstruation)
CTB	ceased to breathe
CTD	carpal tunnel decompression (operation/orthopedics)
CT & DB	cough, turn, and deep breathe
CT ratio	cardiothoracic ratio
Cu	copper
C_u	urea clearance (renal function test) (laboratory/chemistry)
CUC	chronic ulcerative colitis
CUG	cystourethrogram (procedure/urology)
cu. mm.	cubic millimeter
CV	cardiovascular
	cell volume
	central venous (pressure)
	cerebrovascular
	color vision (eye examination)
	corpuscular volume (red blood cells)
CVA	cerebrovascular accident
	costovertebral angle

CVD	cardiovascular disease
cvd.	curved
CVG	coronary vein graft (operation/cardiac)
CVO	conjugate diameter of pelvic inlet (Latin: *conjugata vera obstetrica*)
CVP	central venous pressure
CVR	cardiovascular-respiratory (system)
CVRD	cardiovascular renal disease
CVS	cardiovascular surgery
	cardiovascular system
	clean-voided specimen (procedure/urine culture)
	current vital signs
CW	cardiac work
	chest wall
	clockwise
	crutch walking
CWI	cardiac work index
C.X.	chest x-ray
cx.	cervix (gynecology)
	convex
cyclo.	cyclopropane (anesthetic)
Cysto.	cystoscopy (procedure/urology)

D

D	daughter
	dead
	diopter (eye examination)
	disease

	dispense (on prescriptions)
	distal
	divorced
	dorsal (spines)
d	day
	density
	died (deceased)
	distal
	dose
	duration
	right (Latin: *dextro*)
$D_1, D_2, \ldots$	dorsal vertebrae 1, 2, . . .
DA	degenerative arthritis
	delayed action (with reference to drugs)
	direct agglutination
	dopamine
	ductus arteriosus
DAH	disordered action of the heart
(δ-)ALA	delta-amino-levulinic acid (laboratory/chemistry)
DAPT	direct agglutination pregnancy test (laboratory/serology)
DAT	delayed action tablet (medication orders/prescriptions)
	diphtheria antitoxin
DB	date of birth
db.	decibel
DBI	trade brand of phenformin hydrochloride (medication order)
DBM	diabetic management
DBP	diastolic blood pressure

DC	daily census
	diagnostic code (on records)
	diagonal conjugate
	direct current
	donor's cells
D/C	discontinue
D & C	dilation and curettage (operation/gynecology)
DCA	desoxycorticosterone acetate (medication order)
DCABG	double coronary artery bypass graft
DCG	dynamic electrocardiography
D_{CO}	diffusing capacity for carbon monoxide (pulmonary function test)
DCT	direct Coomb's test (laboratory/blood bank)
	distal convoluted tubule (of kidney)
DD	dependent drainage
	differential diagnosis
	disc diameter (eye examination)
	dry dressing
DDD	degenerative disc disease
DDST	Denver Developmental Screening Test (pediatrics)
DDT	dichlorodiphenyltrichloroethane
DDx.	differential diagnosis
D & E	dilation and evacuation (operation/gynecology)
DEA#	Drug Enforcement Administration number (physician's narcotic number)

dec.	decrease
dec'd.	deceased
decomp.	decompensated (heart disease)
	decomposed
decr.	decreased
def.	defecation
	deficient
	definite
	definition
defic.	deficiency
	deficit
deform.	deformity
deg.	degeneration
	degree
degen.	degeneration (degenerative)
Dem.	Demerol (meperidine hydrochloride) (medication order)
dent.	dental
depr.	depression
deriv.	derivative
	derived
Derm.	dermatology
DES	diethylstilbestrol (medication order)
desat.	desaturated
desc.	descending
determin.	determination
dev.	deviation
devel.	development (developed)

DF	diabetic father
	disseminated foci
DFT$_4$	dialyzable free thyroxine
	(laboratory/endocrinology)
DFU	dead fetus in uterus
DG	diastolic gallop
dgm.	decigram
DHE 45	dihydroergotamine
DHR	delayed hypersensitivity reaction
DHS	duration of hospital stay
D/5 HS	dextrose (5%) in Hartman's solution
	(intravenous solution)
DHSM	dihydrostreptomycin (on culture and
	sensitivity reports)
DHT	dihydrotachysterol (AT-10)
DI	diabetes insipidus
diab.	diabetic (diabetes)
diag.	diagnosis (diagnostic)
	diagonal
diam.	diameter
diath.	diathermy
	(physical therapy)
DIC	disseminated intravascular
	coagulation
diff.	difference
	differential blood count
	(laboratory/hematology)
diff. diag.	differential diagnosis
dig.	digitalis
	(medication order)

Dil.	Dilantin (diphenylhydantoin) (medication order)
dil.	dilute
dilat.	dilatation dilated
DILD	diffuse infiltrative lung disease
diln.	dilution
dim.	diminished
diph.	diphtheria
diph./tet.	diphtheria-tetanus (toxoid) (medication order)
diph. tox.	diphtheria toxoid (medication order)
diph. tox. AP	diphtheria toxoid-alum precipitated (medication order)
DIPJ	distal interphalangeal joint
Dir.	director
dir.	direct directions
dis.	disabled disease distance
disc.	discontinued
disch.	discharge (discharged)
disloc.	dislocation
dism.	dismissed
disp.	dispense (medication orders/prescriptions)
dissd.	dissolved
dissem.	disseminated

dist.	distance
	distill (distilled)
div.	divide
	division
DJD	degenerative joint disease
DK	diet kitchen
dk.	dark
DL	danger list
dl.	deciliter
D_L	diffusing capacity of the lung (pulmonary function test)
DL antibody	Donath-Landsteiner antibody (hemolysin) (laboratory/blood bank)
D_LCO	diffusing capacity of the lung for carbon monoxide (pulmonary function test)
DLE	discoid lupus erythematosus
	disseminated lupus erythematosus
DM	diabetes mellitus
	diabetic mother
	diastolic murmur
DMCT	demethylchlortetracycline (on culture and sensitivity reports)
DMD	Duchenne's muscular dystrophy
DMS	dermatomyositis
DMSO	dimethyl sulfoxide
DN	dicrotic notch
DNA	deoxyribonucleic acid
DNase	deoxyribonuclease
DND	died a natural death

DNK	did not keep (appointment)
DNS	did not show
D5/NSS	dextrose (5%) in normal saline solution (intravenous solution)
DNT	did not test
DO	Doctor of Osteopathy
DOA	dead on arrival
DOB	date of birth doctor's order book
DOC	desoxycorticosterone died of other causes
DOCA	desoxycorticosterone acetate (medication order)
DOD	date of death dead of disease
DOE	dyspnea on exertion
DOI	date of injury
DP	diastolic pressure diffusion pressure diphosphate donor's plasma dorsalis pedis (pulse)
DPC	delayed primary closure
DPD	diffuse pulmonary disease
dp/dt	ratio of change of ventricular pressure to change in time
DPH	diphenylhydantoin (Dilantin) (medication order)
d.p.m.	disintegrations per minute
DPN	diphosphopyridine nucleotide

DPT	diphtheria, pertussis, tetanus (vaccine) (medication order)
DQ	developmental quotient (pediatrics)
DR	diabetic retinopathy diagnostic radiology delivery room dorsal root (spinal nerves)
dr.	dram (medication orders/prescriptions) dressing
DS	dead air space (pulmonary function test) dilute strength (of solution) Down's syndrome (mongolism) dry swallow (medication order)
D/S	dextrose and saline (intravenous solution)
D5/S	dextrose (5%) in saline (intravenous solution)
DSD	dry sterile dressing
dsg.	dressing
DST	daylight saving time dihydrostreptomycin (on culture and sensitivity reports)
DT	distance test (hearing) double tachycardia
DTO	deodorized tincture of opium (medication order)
DTR	deep tendon reflex
DT's	delirium tremens

DU	diagnosis undetermined
	duodenal ulcer
DUB	dysfunctional uterine bleeding
duod.	duodenum
DV	dilute volume (of solution)
DVA	distance visual acuity (eye examination)
DVT	deep vein thrombosis
DW	distilled water (medication orders/prescriptions)
	dry weight
D/W	dextrose in water (intravenous solution)
D5/W (D₅W)	dextrose (5%) in water (intravenous solution)
Dx.	diagnosis
dxd.	discontinued
DXM	dexamethasone
DXT	deep x-ray therapy

E

E	emmetropia (eye examination)
	enema
	enzyme
	eosinophil (on white blood count reports)
	erythromycin (on culture and sensitivity reports)
	esophoria (eye examination)
	expired gas (pulmonary function test)
	eye

E	estrone (laboratory/endocrinology)
E_2	estradiol (17-estradiol) (laboratory/endocrinology)
E_3	estriol (laboratory/endocrinology)
EA	erythrocyte antibody
ea.	each
EAC	erythrocyte antibody complement external auditory canal
EACA	epsilon aminocaproic acid (medication order)
EAM	external auditory meatus
EB	epidermolysis bullosa
EBL	estimated blood loss
EBV	Epstein-Barr virus
EC	enteric-coated (tablets) (medication orders/prescriptions) Escherichia coli (on culture reports) extracellular eyes closed
ECA	ethacrynic acid (diuretic)
ECBV	effective circulating blood volume
ECC	extracorporeal circulation
ECCE	extracapular cataract extraction (operation/ophthalmology)
ECF	extended care facility extracellular fluid
ECFV	extracellular fluid volume
ECG	electrocardiogram (procedure/cardiology)

ECHO	echocardiogram (procedure/cardiology) echoencephalogram (procedure/neurology)
ECHO virus	enterocytopathogenic human orphan virus
ECIB	extracorporeal irradiation of blood
ECL	euglobulin clot lysis (laboratory/hematology)
ECM	extracellular material
E coli	Escherichia coli (laboratory/bacteriology)
EC⊤	enteric-coated tablet (medication orders/prescriptions)
ECV	extracellular volume
ECW	extracellular water
ED	effective dose epidural erythema dose
EDC	estimated date of confinement
EDD	expected date of delivery
EDP	electronic data processing end-diastolic pressure
EDS	Ehlers-Danlos syndrome
EDTA	ethylenediamine tetraacetic acid (medication order)
EDV	end-diastolic volume
EE	end to end (anastomosis) equine encephalitis eye and ear
EEE	Eastern equine encephalitis

EEG	electroencephalogram (procedure/neurology)
EENT	eyes, ears, nose, and throat
EF	ectopic focus ejection fraction extrinsic factor
EFA	essential fatty acids (laboratory/chemistry)
EFE	endocardial fibroelastosis
EFV	extracellular fluid volume
EFVC	expiratory flow-volume curve (pulmonary function test)
EG	esophagogastrectomy (operation/gastrointestinal)
e.g.	for example
EGG	electrogastrogram (procedure/gastroenterology)
EGL	eosinophilic granuloma of the lung
EH	enlarged heart essential hypertension
EHBF	estimated hepatic blood flow
EHL	effective half-life (of radioactive substances)
EHO	extrahepatic obstruction
EHP	extra high potency
EI	enzyme inhibitor
E/I	expiration-inspiration ratio (pulmonary function test)
EIP	extensor indicis proprius
EJB	ectopic junctional beat

EKG	electrocardiogram (procedure/cardiology)
EKY	electrokymogram (procedure/cardiology)
elb.	elbow
elix.	elixir (medication orders/prescriptions)
ELT	euglobulin lysis time
EM	ejection murmur electron microscope emmetropia (eye examination) erythrocyte mass
EMB	ethambutol (tuberculosis therapy)
EMC	encephalomyocarditis
EMF	electromagnetic flowmeter endomyocardial fibrosis
EMG	electromyogram (procedure/physical medicine)
EMT	Emergency Medical Technician
emul.	emulsion (medication orders/prescriptions)
EN	erythema nodosum
Endocrin.	endocrinology
ENG	electronystagmogram (procedure/ophthalmology)
ENT	ears, nose, and throat
EO	eyes open
eo.	eosinophil (on white blood count reports)
EOA	examination, opinion and advice

EOB	emergency observation bed
e.o.d.	every other day
EOG	electrooculogram (procedure/ophthalmology)
EOM	extraocular movements extraocular muscles
eos.	eosinophils (laboratory/hematology)
EP	ectopic pregnancy
EPC	epilepsy
EPEC	enteropathogenic Escherichia coli (laboratory/bacteriology)
Epi.	epinephrine
epith.	epithelial
eq.	equivalent
ER	ejection rate emergency room equivalent roentgen extended release (tablet)
ERA	evoked response audiometry (procedure/otology)
ERBF	effective renal blood flow
ERG	electroretinogram (procedure/ophthalmology)
ERP	effective refractory period
ERV	expiratory reserve volume (pulmonary function test)
ESF	erythropoietic stimulating factor
ESM	ejection systolic murmur
esoph.	esophagus

ESP	end-systolic pressure
	extrasensory perception
ESR	erythrocyte sedimentation rate
	(laboratory/hematology)
ESS	erythrocyte sensitizing substance
ess.	essential
ess. neg.	essentially negative
EST	electroshock therapy
	(procedure/psychiatry)
est.	estimated
ESV	end-systolic volume
ET	ejection time
	endotracheal
	esotropia (eye examination)
	Eustachian tube
et al.	and others (Latin: *et alii*)
ETH	elixir terpin hydrate
	(medication order)
ETH/C	elixir terpin hydrate with codeine
	(medication order)
etiol.	etiology
ETM	erythromycin (on culture and
	sensitivity reports)
ETOH	ethyl alcohol (whiskey)
ETP	entire treatment period
ETR	effective thyroxine ratio
	(nuclear medicine)
EU	Ehrlich units (urobilinogen)
	emergency unit
	enzyme units

EUA	examination under anesthetic (procedure/gynecology)
EV	extravascular
eval.	evaluate (evaluation)
EWB	estrogen withdrawal bleeding
ex.	examined example
exam.	examination
exc.	except excision
exp.	expected expectorated expired
expir.	expiration expiratory
exp. lap.	exploratory laparotomy (operation/abdominal)
expt.	expectorant (medication orders/prescriptions)
ext.	extend extension extensor external extract extremity

F

F	Fahrenheit female gas concentration

f	focal frequency from
F_1	first filial generation
F_2	second filial generation
FA	fatty acid first aid folic acid
fam. doc.	family doctor
fam. phys.	family physician
FANA	fluorescent antinuclear antibodies (laboratory/chemistry)
FB	finger breadth foreign body
FBP	femoral blood pressure fibrin breakdown products (laboratory/coagulation)
FBS	fasting blood sugar (laboratory/chemistry)
FC	finger counting (eye examination)
F. cath.	Foley catheter
FD	fatal dose focal distance (eye examination) foot drape forceps delivery (obstetrics)
FDA	Food and Drug Administration
FDP	fibrin degradation product (laboratory/coagulation)
Fe	iron (Latin: *ferrum*)
^{59}Fe	radioactive iron (nuclear medicine)

feb. agglut.	febrile agglutinin (laboratory/serology)
feb. dur.	while the fever lasts (Latin: *febre durante*)
FECG	fetal electrocardiogram (procedure/obstetrics)
FECVC	functional extracellular fluid volume
Fe def.	iron deficiency (anemia)
FEF	forced expiratory flow (pulmonary function test)
fem.	female (feminine) femoral
FES	forced expiratory spirogram (pulmonary function test)
FET	forced expiratory time (pulmonary function test)
FETS	forced expiratory time, in seconds (pulmonary function test)
FEV	forced expiratory volume (pulmonary function test)
FEV_1	forced expiratory volume in one second (pulmonary function test)
FF	fat free (diet) finger to finger (neurological examination) flat feet force fluids (diet order)
FFA	free fatty acids (laboratory/chemistry)

FFP	fresh frozen plasma
FH	family history
	fetal head
	fetal heart
FHR	fetal heart rate
FHS	fetal heart sounds
F Hx.	family history
fib.	fibrillation
fibrin.	fibrinogen (laboratory/coagulation)
FICO$_2$	concentration of carbon dioxide in inspired gas (respiratory therapy)
FIF	forced inspiratory flow (pulmonary function test)
fig.	figure
filt.	filter
FIO$_2$	concentration of oxygen in inspired gas (respiratory therapy)
fist.	fistula
FJN	familial juvenile nephrophthisis
fl.	fluid
FLB	funny looking beat (ECG)
FLC	funny looking child (pediatrics)
fld.	fluid
fld. ext.	fluid extract (medication orders/prescriptions)
fl. dr.	fluid dram (medication orders/prescriptions)

flex.	flexion
FLK	funny looking kid (pediatrics)
fl. oz.	fluid ounce (medication orders/prescriptions)
FLSA	follicular lymphosarcoma
fluor.	fluorescent fluoroscopy (procedure/radiology)
fl. up	flare up follow up
FM	flow meter nitrofurantoin (on culture and sensitivity reports)
FME	full mouth extraction (operation/oral surgery)
FMF	familial Mediterranean fever
FMG	foreign medical graduate
FMS	fat-mobilizing substances
FN	false-negative finger to nose (neurological examination)
FO	foramen ovale (heart) fronto-occipital
FOD	free of disease
for. body	foreign body
FOW	fenestration oval window (operation/otology)
FP	false-positive family planning flat plate (x-ray/abdomen) frozen plasma

FR	French (catheter gauge)
fract.	fracture
FRC	functional reserve capacity (of lungs) (pulmonary function test) functional residual capacity (of lungs) (pulmonary function test)
freq.	frequent (frequency)
FRF	follicle-stimulating hormone releasing factor (laboratory/endocrinology)
frict.	friction (rub)
FROM	full range-of-motion
FRP	functional refractory period
FS	full and soft (diet order)
FSF	fibrin stabilizing factor (Factor XIII) (laboratory/coagulation)
FSH	follicle-stimulating hormone (laboratory/endocrinology)
FT	family therapy fibrous tissue follow through (after barium meal) (x-ray/intestines) full term (obstetrics)
FT_4	free thyroxine (laboratory/endocrinology)
ft.	feet foot

FTA	fluorescent treponemal antibodies (syphilis) (laboratory/serology)
FTA-Abs	fluorescent treponemal antibody absorption (test) (laboratory/serology)
FTG	full thickness graft (operation/plastic surgery)
FTI	free thyroxine index (laboratory/endocrinology)
FTND	full term normal delivery
FTT	failure to thrive
FU	fecal urobilinogen (laboratory/chemistry)
5-FU	5-fluorouracil (cancer chemotherapy)
f/u	follow up
FUO	fever of unknown origin
FV	fluid volume
FVC	forced vital capacity (pulmonary function test)
FVE	forced volume, expiratory (pulmonary function test)
FWB	full weight bearing
FW reaction	Felix-Weil reaction (laboratory/serology)
Fx.	fracture
Fx. BB	fracture of both bones

G

G	gas
	globulin
	glucose
	good
	gravida
	green
g	acceleration due to gravity
	gram
GA	gastric analysis
	(procedure/gastroenterology)
	general anesthesia
	general appearance
	gestational age
^{67}Ga	radioactive gallium
	(nuclear medicine)
g.a.	ginger ale
	(diet order)
ga.	gauge (of needles)
gal.	gallon
garg.	gargle
GB	gallbladder
	goofball (barbiturate)
	Guillain-Barré (syndrome)
GBA	ganglionic-blocking agent
GBM	glomerular basement membrane
GBS	gallbladder series
	(x-ray/gallbladder)
G.B. series	gallbladder series
	(x-ray/gallbladder)

GC	gas chromotography
	gonococcus (gonorrhea)
	granular casts (urine)
g-cal.	gram-calorie
g-cm.	gram-centimeter
gd.	good
GDH	gonadotropic hormone
GE	gastroenterology
	gastroenterostomy
	(operation/stomach)
G/E	granulocyte-erythroid ratio
	(laboratory/hematology)
gen.	general
Ger.	geriatrics
GF	glomerular filtration
	gluten-free
	(diet order)
	grandfather
GFD	gluten-free diet
	(diet order)
GFR	glomerular filtration rate
GG	gamma globulin
	(medication order)
GGE	generalized glandular enlargement
GG or S	glands, goiter, or stiffness
GH	growth hormone
	(laboratory/endocrinology)
GHD	growth hormone deficiency
GHRF	growth hormone releasing factor
	(laboratory/endocrinology)

GI	gastrointestinal
	globin insulin
GIK	glucose, insulin, and potassium (intravenous solution)
GIS	gastrointestinal series (x-ray/stomach)
	gastrointestinal system
G.I. series	gastrointestinal series (x-ray/stomach)
GIT	gastrointestinal tract
gl.	gland
GLC	gas-liquid chromatography
glob.	globulin (laboratory/chemistry)
GLPP	glucose, post prandial (laboratory/chemistry)
gluc.	glucose (laboratory/chemistry)
GM	gastric mucosa
	gentamicin (on culture and sensitivity reports)
	grandmother
	grand multiparity
Gm. (gm.)	gram
Gm. −	gram stain negative (on bacteriology reports)
Gm. +	gram stain positive (on bacteriology reports)
Gm.%	grams per hundred milliliters
gm.-m	gram-meter
GM seizure	grand mal seizure

GN	glomerulonephritis Graduate Nurse
GNID	gram-negative intracellular diplococci
G/NS	glucose in normal saline (intravenous solution)
GOE	gas, oxygen, ether (anesthesia)
GP	general paresis general practitioner
G6PD	glucose-6-phosphate dehydrogenase (laboratory/chemistry)
GPKA	guinea pig kidney absorption test (laboratory/serology)
GR	gastric resection (operation/stomach)
gr.	grain (medication orders/prescriptions) gravity
grad.	gradient gradually graduated
gran.	granular
grav.	gravida (pregnancy) gravity
grav. †	primagravida (first pregnancy)
grav. † /Ab. †	one pregnancy, one abortion
grav. ō	no pregnancies
GRF	gonadotropin-releasing factor (laboratory/endocrinology)
GS	general surgery

G/S	glucose and saline (intravenous solution)
GSC	gas-solid chromatography
GSD	glycogen storage disease
GSE	gluten-sensitive enteropathy
GSR	galvanic skin response
GSW	gunshot wound
GT	genetic therapy glucose tolerance
GTH	gonadotropic hormone (laboratory/endocrinology)
GTT	glucose tolerance test (diabetes detection) (laboratory/chemistry)
gtts.	drops (Latin: *guttae*) (medication orders/prescriptions)
GU	gastric ulcer genitourinary gonococcal urethritis
GUS	genitourinary system
GV	gentian violet (dye) (medication order)
GVHR	graft versus host reaction
G/W	glucose in water (intravenous solution)
GWE	glycerin and water enema (procedure/enema)
GXT	graded exercise test (procedure/cardiology)
Gyn.	gynecology

H

H	heroin horizontal hormone human husband hydrogen hypermetropia (eye examination)
h	hour
Ⓗ	hypodermic injection (medication order)
H+	hydrogen ion
HA	headache hearing aid hemagglutination hemolytic anemia heterophile antibody (infectious mononucleosis) (laboratory/serology) hospital admission
Ha.	absolute hypermetropia (eye examination)
HAA	hepatitis associated antigen (Australia antigen) (laboratory/serology)
HAE	hereditary angioneurotic edema
HAI	hemagglutination inhibition (laboratory/hematology)
HASHD	hypertensive arteriosclerotic heart disease
HB	heart block (electrocardiogram) hold breakfast

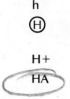

Hb. (Hgb.)	hemoglobin (laboratory/hematology)
HBAg	hepatitis B antigen (laboratory/virology)
HB/BW	hold breakfast for blood work
HBD	alpha-hydroxybutyric dehydrogenase (laboratory/chemistry)
HBDH	hydroxybutyric dehydrogenase (laboratory/chemistry)
HBE	His bundle electrogram (procedure/cardiology)
HBF	hepatic blood flow
Hb-F	fetal hemoglobin (laboratory/hematology)
HBIG	hepatitis B immunoglobulin
HBO	hyperbaric oxygen
HBP	high blood pressure
HBS	hyperkinetic behavior syndrome
HBsAg	hepatitis B surface antigen (laboratory/virology)
HBV	hepatitis B virus
HC	home care house call Huntington's chorea hyaline casts (urine) hydrocortisone
HCC	history of chief complaint hydroxycholecalciferol (Vitamin D)
HCG	human chorionic gonadotropin (laboratory/endocrinology)

HCl	hydrochloric acid
	hydrochloride
HCO₃	bicarbonate
	(laboratory/chemistry)
HCSM	human chorionic
	somatomammotropin
	(laboratory/endocrinology)
Hct. (hct.)	hematocrit
	(laboratory/hematology)
HCTZ	hydrochlorothiazide
HCU	homocystinuria
HCVD	hypertensive cardiovascular disease
HD	Hansen's disease (leprosy)
	hearing distance
	heart disease
	Hodgkin's disease
HDBH	hydroxybutyric dehydrogenase
	(laboratory/chemistry)
HDL	high density lipoproteins
	(laboratory/chemistry)
HDN	hemolytic disease of the newborn
HDS	herniated disc syndrome
HDW	hearing distance with watch
H & E	hematoxylin and eosin (stain)
	heredity and environment
HEAT	human erythrocyte agglutination test
	(laboratory/hematology)
HEENT	head, eyes, ears, nose, throat
HEK	human embryonic kidney
HEL	human embryonic lung
Hematol.	hematology

HEV	human enteric virus
HF	Hageman factor (laboratory/coagulation)
	hay fever
	heart failure
	high frequency
HFI	hereditary fructose intolerance
Hg	mercury (Latin: *hydrargyrum*)
Hgb.	hemoglobin (laboratory/hematology)
HGF	hyperglycemic glycogenolytic factor
Hg-F	fetal hemoglobin (laboratory/hematology)
HGG	human gamma globulin
HGH	human growth hormone (laboratory/endocrinology)
HH	hiatal hernia
H & H	hemoglobin and hematocrit (laboratory/hematology)
HHA	hereditary hemolytic anemia
HHD	hypertensive heart disease
HHE	hemiconvulsions, hemiplegia, epilepsy
HHNK	hyperglycemic hyperosmolar nonketotic coma
HHT	hereditary hemorrhagic telangiectasia
HI	hemagglutination inhibition (laboratory/hematology)
HIA	hemagglutination inhibition antibody (laboratory/hematology)

5-HIAA	5-hydroxyindoleacetic acid (laboratory/chemistry)
HID	hyperkinetic impulse disorder
HJ bodies	Howell-Jolly bodies
HJ reflex	hepatojugular reflex
H-K	heel to knee
HL	half-life (of a radioactive element) harelip hearing loss hypermetropia, latent (eye examination)
H & L	heart and lungs
HLA	human lymphocyte antibody (laboratory/serology)
HLD	herniated lumbar disc
HLDH	heat stable lactic dehydrogenase (laboratory/chemistry)
HLH	human luteinizing hormone (laboratory/endocrinology)
HLR	heart-lung resuscitation
HLV	herpes-like virus
HM	hand movements hydantidiform mole hypermetropia, manifest (eye examination)
HMD	hyaline membrane disease
HMG	human menopausal gonadotropin (laboratory/endocrinology)
HMO	Health Maintenance Organization
HMP	hot moist packs
HN	Head Nurse

HN_2	nitrogen mustard (medication order)
H & N	head and neck
HNP	herniated nucleus pulposus
HNSHA	hereditary nonspherocytic hemolytic anemia
HNV	has not voided
HO	House Officer (intern or resident physician) hyperbaric oxygen
h/o	history of
H_2O	water
H_2O_2	hydrogen peroxide (medication order)
HOB	head of bed
HOP	high oxygen pressure (respiratory therapy)
hosp.	hospital
HP	high potency high power high protein (diet order) hot pack (pad) House Physician hydrostatic pressure
Hp	hemiplegia
H & P	history and physical
HPA	hypothalamic-pituitary-adrenal (axis)
HPE	history and physical examination
h.p.f.	per high-power field (microscopy)

HPFH	hereditary persistence of fetal hemoglobin
HPG	human pituitary gonadotropin (laboratory/endocrinology)
HPI	history of present illness
HPL	human placental lactogen (laboratory/endocrinology)
HPO	high pressure oxygen (respiratory therapy)
HPS	high protein supplement (diet order) hypertrophic pyloric stenosis
HPT	hyperparathyroidism
HPVD	hypertensive pulmonary vascular disease
HR	heart rate hospital record
hr.	hour
H & R	hysterectomy and radiation (operation/gynecology)
HRIG	human rabies immune globulin (medication order)
HS	half strength Hartman's solution (intravenous solution) heart sounds heat stable hereditary spherocytosis herpes simplex horse serum Hurler's syndrome

h.s.	at bedtime (Latin: *hora somni*) (medication orders/prescriptions)
	hour of sleep
HSA	human serum albumin (medication order)
HSG	hysterosalpingogram (procedure/gynecology)
HSV	herpes simplex virus
HT	hearing test
	hydrotherapy (physical therapy)
	hypermetropia, total (eye examination)
	hypodermic tablet
ht.	heart
	height
5-HT	5-hydroxytryptamine (serotonin) (laboratory/endocrinology)
HTN	hypertension
HTV	herpes-type virus
HUS	hemolytic uremic syndrome
husb.	husband
HV	hepatic vein
	herpes virus
	hyperventilation
H & V	hemigastrectomy and vagotomy (operation/stomach)
HVA	homovanillic acid (laboratory/endocrinology)
HVD	hypertensive vascular disease
HW	housewife

hwb	hot water bottle
Hx.	history
Hy.	hypermetropia (eye examination)
hypo.	hypochromasia (red blood cells)
	hypodermic injection
	(medication order)
hys.	hysteria
hyst.	hysterectomy
	(operation/gynecology)
HZ	herpes zoster
Hz.	Hertz (electrical measurement)

I

I	index
	inhibitor
	iodine
^{131}I	radioactive iodine
	(nuclear medicine)
IA	incidental appendectomy
	(operation/abdominal)
	internal auditory (ear)
	intraarterial (blood pressure)
	intraarticular (injection)
IABC	intraaortic balloon counterpulsation
	(procedure/cardiology)
IABP	intraaortic balloon pumping
	(procedure/cardiology)
IAC	internal auditory canal
IADHS	inappropriate antidiuretic hormone
	syndrome

IAM	internal auditory meatus
IAS	intra-amniotic saline infusion (procedure/gynecology)
IASD	intraatrial septal defect (heart)
IB	inclusion body
IBC	iron-binding capacity (laboratory/chemistry)
IBI	intermittent bladder irrigation (procedure/urology)
IC	inspiratory capacity (pulmonary function test)
	intensive care
	intercostal
	intermediate care
	interstitial cells
	intracavitary
	intracellular
	intracerebral
	intracranial
	intracutaneous (injection site)
	irritable colon
	isovolumic contraction (heart)
ICA	intracranial aneurysm
ICC	intensive coronary care
ICCE	intracapsular cataract extraction (operation/ophthalmology)
ICCEc̄PI	intracapsular cataract extraction with peripheral iridectomy (operation/ophthalmology)
ICCU	intensive coronary care unit
ICDH	isocitric dehydrogenase (laboratory/chemistry)

ICF	intensive care facility
	intermediate care facility
	intracellular fluid
ICG	indocyanine green (dye)
ICH	intracerebral hemorrhage
ICM	intercostal margin
ICP	intracranial pressure
ICS	intercostal space
ICSH	interstitial cell-stimulating hormone (laboratory/endocrinology)
ICT	indirect Coombs' test (laboratory/blood bank)
	isovolumic contraction time (heart)
ict.	icterus (jaundice)
ict. ind.	icterus index (laboratory/chemistry)
ICU	intensive care unit
ICW	intracellular water
ID	identification
	infant deaths
	infectious disease
	initial diagnosis
	initial dose
	internal diameter
	intradermal (injection site)
id.	the same (Latin: *idem*)
I & D	incision and drainage (operation/skin)
IDA	iron deficiency anemia
IDI	induction-delivery interval
IDM	infant of diabetic mother

IDS	immunity deficiency state
IDVC	indwelling venous catheter
I/E	inspiratory-expiratory ratio (pulmonary function test)
IEMG	integrated electromyogram (procedure/physical medicine)
IEOP	immunoelectro-osmophoresis
IEP	immunoelectrophoresis
IF	immunofluorescence interstitial fluid intrinsic factor
IFA	indirect fluorescent antibody
IFC	intrinsic factor concentrate
IFR	inspiratory flow rate (respiratory therapy)
IFV	intracellular fluid volume
IG	immune globulin intragastric
Ig	immunoglobulin (laboratory/serology) *Types of immunoglobulins:* IgA (gamma A) IgD (gamma D) IgE (gamma E) IgG (gamma G) IgM (gamma M)
IGDM	infant of gestational diabetic mother
IH	infectious hepatitis
IHA	indirect hemagglutination (laboratory/serology)
IHBT	incompatible hemolytic blood transfusion

IHD	ischemic heart disease
IHO	idiopathic hypertrophic osteoarthropathy
IHR	intrinsic heart rate
IHSA	iodinated human serum albumin
[^{131}I] HSA	human serum albumin tagged with radioiodine (nuclear medicine)
IHSS	idiopathic hypertrophic subaortic stenosis
IIF	indirect immunofluorescent
ILA	insulin-like activity
ILBW	infant, low birth weight
ILD	ischemic leg disease ischemic limb disease
IM	infectious mononucleosis internal medicine intramedullary intramuscular (injection site)
IMA	internal mammary artery (implant) (operation/heart)
IMB	intermenstrual bleeding
IMBC	indirect maximum breathing capacity (pulmonary function test)
IMH	idiopathic myocardial hypertrophy
IMI	inferior myocardial infarction
immun.	immunology
imp.	important impression improved
IMR	infant mortality rate

IMV	intermittent mechanical ventilation (respiratory therapy)
IN	intranasal
In.	insulin
in.	inch
inac.	inactive
inc.	incision incurred
incl.	include (including)
incr.	increased (increasing)
IND	investigational new drug
ind.	independent indirect
INDM	infant of nondiabetic mother
inf.	infant infantile infected infection inferior infusion
infec. dis.	infectious disease
Inf. MI	inferior wall myocardial infarction
info.	information
ing.	inguinal
INH	isonicotinic acid hydrazide (isoniazid) (medication order)
inh.	inhalation
inj.	inject (injection) injury

inoc.	inoculate (inoculation)
INPV	intermittent negative-pressure assisted ventilation (respiratory therapy)
INS	idiopathic nephrotic syndrome
ins.	insurance
inspir.	inspiration (inspiratory)
int.	internal
Int. Med.	internal medicine
IO	inferior oblique (muscle) internal os (cervix) intestinal obstruction intraocular
I & O	intake and output
IOFB	intraocular foreign body
IOP	intraocular pressure
IP	incubation period interphalangeal (joint) intraperitoneal (injection site) isoelectric point
IPG	impedance plethysmography (procedure/cardiology)
IPH	idiopathic pulmonary hemosiderosis
IPP	intermittent positive pressure (respiratory therapy)
IPPB	intermittent positive pressure breathing (respiratory therapy)
IPPI	interruption of pregnancy for psychiatric indication

IPPO	intermittent positive pressure inflation with oxygen (respiratory therapy)
IPPV	intermittent positive pressure ventilation (respiratory therapy)
IPU	inpatient unit
IPV	inactivated poliomyelitis vaccine
IQ	intelligence quotient
IR	immunoreactive inferior rectus (muscle) infra-red rays (procedure/physical medicine)
IRBBB	incomplete right bundle branch block (ECG)
IRDS	idiopathic respiratory distress syndrome
irr.	irradiation
irrig.	irrigation
IRS	infra-red spectrophotometry
IRV	inspiratory reserve volume (pulmonary function test)
IS	immune serum *in situ* (in original place) intercostal space interspace intraspinal
ISA	intrinsic sympathomimetic activity
ISC	interstitial cells
ISF	interstitial fluid

ISG	immune serum globulin (medication order)
ISH	icteric serum hepatitis
IST	insulin sensitivity test (procedure/endocrinology) insulin shock therapy (procedure/psychiatry)
ISW	interstitial water
IT	inhalation therapy (respiratory therapy) intertuberous (pelvic diameter) intradermal test intrathoracic intratracheal intratracheal tube
Ith.	intrathecal (intraspinal)
ITP	idiopathic thrombocytopenic purpura
ITT	insulin tolerance test (procedure/endocrinology)
IU	international unit intrauterine
IUCD	intrauterine contraceptive device
IUD	intrauterine death intrauterine device
IU/L	international units per liter
IV	interventricular (heart) intervertebral intravascular intravenous
IVC	inferior vena cava
IVCC	intravascular consumption coagulopathy

IVCD	intraventricular conduction defect (ECG)
IVCP	Inferior vena cava pressure
IVCV	inferior venacavography (x-ray/vascular)
IVD	intervertebral disc
IVF	intravascular fluid
IVGTT	intravenous glucose tolerance test (procedure/endocrinology)
IVH	intraventricular hemorrhage (brain)
IVP	intravenous push (dose) intravenous pyelogram (x-ray/kidneys)
IVPB	intravenous piggypack (infusion) (intravenous therapy)
IVSD	intraventricular septal defect (heart)
IVU	intravenous urography (x-ray/kidneys)
IWMI	inferior wall myocardial infarction

J

J	Jewish joint joule (electrical measurement)
jaund.	jaundice
jc.	juice (diet order)
jct.	junction
jej.	jejunum

JGA	juxtaglomerular apparatus (kidney)
JGC	juxtaglomerular cell (kidney)
JJ	jaw jerk (neurologic examination)
JND	just noticeable difference
JOB	juvenile onset diabetes
JPB	junctional premature beat
JPC	junctional premature contraction
JR	junctional rhythm
jt.	joint
juve.	juvenile
JV	jugular vein
JVD	jugular venous distention
JVP	jugular venous pulse
JVPT	jugular venous pulse tracing (procedure/cardiology)

K

K	absolute zero (temperature) a thousand kanamycin (on culture and sensitivity reports) kilogram potassium (Latin: *kalium*) (laboratory/chemistry)
k	constant
17K	17-ketosteroid excretion (laboratory/endocrinology)
KA	ketoacidosis King-Armstrong (units)

KB	ketone bodies (laboratory/urine)
kc.	kilocycle (electrical measurement)
kcal.	kilocalorie
KCG	kinetocardiogram (procedure/cardiology)
KCl	potassium chloride (medication orders/prescriptions)
kc/s	kilocycles per second
K_e	exchangeable body potassium
keto.	17-ketosteroid (laboratory/endocrinology)
kev.	kiloelectron volts
KFAB	kidney-fixing antibody
KFS	Klippel-Feil syndrome
kg.	kilogram
kg/cal	kilogram-calorie
KGS	ketogenic steroid (laboratory/endocrinology)
kilo	a thousand grams (kilogram)
KJ	knee jerk (neurologic examination)
KK	knee kick (neurologic examination)
kl.	kiloliter
K.L. bac.	Klebs-Loeffler bacillus (on bacteriology reports)
Klebs	Klebsiella (on bacteriology reports)
KLS	kidney, liver, spleen
KM	kanamycin (on culture and sensitivity reports)

km.	kilometer
km/s	kilometers per second
KMV	killed measles-virus vaccine
kn.	knee
K/O	keep open
KOH	potassium hydroxide
KP	keratitis punctata (eye examination)
KRP	Krebs-Ringer phosphate (intravenous solution)
KS	ketosteroid (laboratory/endocrinology)
	Klinefelter's syndrome
	Kveim-Seltzback (test)
KUB	kidney, ureter, bladder (x-ray/urology)
kva.	kilovolt-ampere
KVO	keep vein open (intravenous therapy)
KW	Keith-Wagener (eyeground findings)
	Kimmelstiel-Wilson (disease)
KWB	Keith, Wagener, Barker classification of eyeground findings

L

L	left
	length
	liter
	lower
	lumbar
Ⓛ	left

l	long
L₁, L₂, . . .	lumbar vertebrae 1, 2, . . .
LA	lactic acid (laboratory/chemistry)
	large amount
	left arm
	left atrium
	local anesthesia
	long-acting (drug)
L & A	light and accommodation (eye examination)
lab.	laboratory
lac.	laceration
LAD	left anterior descending (coronary artery)
	left axis deviation
LAE	left atrial enlargement
LAF	laminar air flow
LAH	left anterior hemiblock (ECG)
LAIT	latex agglutination inhibition test (laboratory/serology)
LAM	late ambulatory monitoring
LAO	left anterior oblique
LAP	left atrial pressure
	leukocyte alkaline phosphatase (laboratory/hematology)
lap.	laparoscopy (procedure/abdominal)
	laparotomy (operation/abdominal)
Laryng.	laryngology

LASER	light amplification by stimulated emission of radiation (radiation therapy)
LAT	left anterior thigh (injection site)
lat.	lateral
LATS	long-acting thyroid stimulator
lax.	laxative (medication order)
LB	left buttock (injection site)
	live birth
	loose body
	low back
lb.	pound (Latin: *libra*)
LBBB	left bundle branch block (ECG)
LBCD	left border cardiac dullness
LBD	left border of dullness
LBM	lean body mass
	loose bowel movement
LBP	low back pain
	low blood pressure
LBW	low birth weight
LC	late clamped (umbilical cord)
	living children
LCA	left coronary artery
LCFA	long-chain fatty acid
LCL	lymphocytic lymphosarcoma
LCM	left costal margin
	lymphocytic choriomeningitis
LCT	long-chain triglyceride

LD	left deltoid (injection site)
	light difference (eye examination)
	longitudinal diameter
	low density
L & D	labor and delivery
LD_{50}	median lethal dose
L-D bodies	Leishman-Donovan bodies (laboratory/bacteriology)
LDD	light-dark discrimination (eye examination)
LDH	lactic dehydrogenase (laboratory/chemistry)
LDL	low density lipoproteins (laboratory/chemistry)
L-dopa	levodopa (medication order)
LE	lower extremity
	lupus erythematosus
LED	lupus erythematosus disseminatus
LE prep.	lupus erythematosus preparation (laboratory/hematology)
leuko.	leukocytes (laboratory/hematology)
LF	latex fixation (test) (laboratory/serology)
	low forceps (delivery)
LFA	left femoral artery
	left frontoanterior (fetal position)
LFD	lactose free diet (diet order)
	low fat diet (diet order)
	low forceps delivery

LFP	left frontoposterior (fetal position)
LFS	liver function series (laboratory/chemistry)
LFT	latex flocculation test (laboratory/serology) left frontotransverse (fetal position) liver function test
LG	left gluteus (injection site) lymph glands
lg.	large
LGB	Landry-Guillain-Barré (syndrome)
LGV	lymphogranuloma venereum
LH	left hand luteinizing hormone (laboratory/endocrinology)
LHF	left heart failure
LHL	left hepatic lobe
LHRF	luteinizing hormone releasing factor
Li.	lithium
LIF	left iliac fossa (injection site)
lig.	ligament
lin.	linear liniment (medication orders/prescriptions)
LIQ	lower inner quadrant
liq.	liquid (diet order) liquor
LK	left kidney
LKS	liver, kidney, spleen

LL	left leg
	left lower
	left lung
	lower lid
	lower lobe
LLB	long leg brace (orthopedics)
LLE	left lower extremity
LLL	left lower lobe (lung)
LLM	localized leukocyte mobilization
LLQ	left lower quadrant
LLT	left lateral thigh (injection site)
LM	light microscopy
	longitudinal muscle
	lower motor (neuron)
LMA	left mentoanterior (fetal position)
LMD	local medical doctor
	low molecular weight dextran (intravenous solution)
L/min.	liters per minute
L/min/m²	liters per minute per square meter
LML	left mediolateral (episiotomy) (operation/obstetrics)
LMP	last menstrual period
	left mentoposterior (fetal position)
LMT	left mentotransverse (fetal position)
LN	lymph node
LNMP	last normal menstrual period
LOA	leave of absence
	left occiput anterior (fetal position)
LOM	limitation of motion
	loss of motion

LOP	leave on pass
	left occiput posterior (fetal position)
LOQ	lower outer quadrant
LOT	left occiput transverse (fetal position)
lot.	lotion
	(medication orders/prescriptions)
LOWBI	low birth weight infant
LP	latent period
	leukocyte-poor
	light perception (eye examination)
	lipoprotein
	low power (microscopy)
	low pressure
	low protein
	(diet order)
	lumbar puncture
	(procedure/neurology)
LPA	left pulmonary artery
LPE	lipoprotein electrophoresis
	(laboratory/chemistry)
LPF	low power field (microscopy)
LPH	left posterior hemiblock (ECG)
LPL	lipoprotein lipase
LPN	Licensed Practical Nurse
LPO	light perception only
	(eye examination)
L/P ratio	lactate pyruvate ratio
	(laboratory/endocrinology)
LPV	left pulmonary veins
LR	labor room
L & R	left and right

L→R	left to right
LRS	lactated Ringer's solution (intravenous solution)
LR	lower respiratory tract
LS	left side liver and spleen lumbosacral lymphosarcoma
LSA	left sacrum anterior (fetal position)
LSA/RCS	lymphosarcoma-reticulum cell sarcoma
LSB	left sternal border
LSCA	left scapuloanterior (fetal position)
LSCP	left scapuloposterior (fetal position)
LSD	lysergic acid diethylamide
LSK	liver, spleen, kidneys
LSM	late systolic murmur
LSP	left sacrum posterior (fetal position)
L/S ratio	lecithin to sphingomyelin ratio (in amniotic fluid) (laboratory/chemistry)
LST	left sacrum transverse (fetal position)
LSV	left subclavian vein
LT	left thigh Levin tube (for gastrointestinal suction) levothyroxine long term
lt.	left light

LTB	laryngo-tracheal bronchitis
LTH	lactogenic hormone
	luteotrophic hormone
lt. lat.	left lateral
LU	left upper
L & U	lower and upper
LUE	left upper extremity
LUL	left upper lobe (lung)
LUQ	left upper quadrant
LV	left ventricle
LVDP	left ventricular diastolic pressure
LVE	left ventricular enlargement
LVEDP	left ventricular end-diastolic pressure
LVEDV	left ventricular end-diastolic volume
LVET	left ventricular ejection time
LVF	left ventricular failure
LVH	left ventricular hypertrophy
LVN	Licensed Vocational Nurse
LVP	left ventricular pressure
LVSV	left ventricular stroke volume
LVSW	left ventricular stroke work
LVW	left ventricular work
LVWI	left ventricular work index
L & W	living and well
LWCT	Lee-White clotting time
lymphs	lymphocytes
	(laboratory/hematology)
lytes	electrolytes
	(laboratory/chemistry)

M

M	male
	married
	mass
	Micrococcus (on bacteriology reports)
	Microsporum (on bacteriology reports)
	mix (prescriptions)
	monocyte (on white blood counts)
	month
	mother
	muscle
	Mycobacterium (on bacteriology reports)
	Mycoplasma (on bacteriology reports)
	myopia (eye examination)
m	meter
	minim (1/60 of a dram, or one drop) (medication orders/prescriptions)
	minute
M_1	mitral first heart sound
M_2	mitral second heart sound
M^2	square meters (of body surface)
MA	mental age
ma.	milliampere (electrical measurement)
MABP	mean arterial blood pressure
mac.	macerate
mag.	large (Latin: *magnus*)
mag. cit.	magnesium citrate (laxative) (medication order)
magnif.	magnification

malig.	malignant
M+AM	compound myopic astigmatism
mam.	milliampere minute
mand.	mandible
manifest	manifestation
manip.	manipulation
MAO	monoamine oxidase
MAOI	monoamine oxidase inhibitor
MAP	mean aortic pressure
	mean arterial pressure
	muscle action potential (procedure/physical medicine)
MAS	meconium aspiration syndrome
mas.	milliampere second
masc.	masculine
MASER	microwave amplification by stimulated emission of radiation (radiation therapy)
MA tube	Miller-Abbott tube (for gastrointestinal suction)
max.	maximum (maximal)
MB	methylene blue (dye)
6MB	six meal bland diet (diet order)
MBC	maximum breathing capacity (pulmonary function test)
	minimal bactericidal concentration
MBD	minimal brain dysfunction
MBF	myocardial blood flow
MBL	minimal bactericidal level

MBP	mean blood pressure
MC	mast cell (on blood smear)
	maximum concentration
	metacarpal (joint)
M & C	morphine and cocaine (drug addiction)
mC	millicurie (radioactivity measurement)
MCB	membranous cytoplasmic bodies
McB. pt.	McBurney's point
MCC	mean corpuscular hemoglobin concentration (laboratory/hematology)
MCD	mean cell diameter
	mean corpuscular diameter (laboratory/hematology)
mcg.	microgram
MCH	Maternal and Child Health
	mean corpuscular hemoglobin (laboratory/hematology)
MCHC	mean corpuscular hemoglobin concentration (laboratory/hematology)
MCI	mean cardiac index
MCL	midclavicular line
	midcostal line
	modified chest lead (ECG)
MCLS	mucocutaneous lymph node syndrome
MCP	metacarpal phalangeal (joint)
MCR	metabolic clearance rate
mc/s	megacycles per second

MCT	mean circulation time
	mean corpuscular thickness (laboratory/hematology)
MCU	maximum care unit
mcU	microunit (on laboratory reports)
MCV	mean corpuscular volume (laboratory/hematology)
MD	manic depressive (psychiatry)
	mean deviation
	medical doctor
	mentally deficient
	minimum dosage
	mitral disease (cardiology)
	movement disorder (neurology)
	muscular dystrophy
	myocardial disease (cardiology)
MDA	right mentoanterior (fetal position)
MDD	mean daily dose
MDF	myocardial depressant factor
MDM	mid-diastolic murmur
MDP	right mentoposterior (fetal position)
MDR	minimum daily requirement
MDT	right mentotransverse (fetal position)
MDUO	myocardial disease of unknown origin
MDV	multiple dose vial (prescriptions)
MDY	month, date, year
ME	Medical Examiner
	middle ear
M/E	myeloid-erythroid ratio (laboratory/hematology)

MEA	multiple endocrine adenomatosis
meas.	measure (measurement)
MEC	minimum effective concentration
MED	median erythrocyte diameter (laboratory/hematology) minimal effective dose minimal erythema dose (x-ray therapy)
med.	medial median medical medicine medium (bacteriology)
meds.	medications (medicines)
MEF	maximal expiratory flow (pulmonary function test)
MEFR	maximum expiratory flow rate (pulmonary function test)
memb.	membrane
ment.	mental
MEP	mean effective pressure meperidine (Demerol)
mEq.	milliequivalent (on chemistry reports)
MER	mean ejection rate
MES	maximal electroshock seizure
Mesc.	mescaline
met.	metastatic (metastasis)
metab.	metabolism (metabolic)
metas.	metastatic (metastasis)
met. series	metastatic series (x-ray/chest, bones, skull)

mev.	million electron volts
MF	Millipore filter (for intravenous therapy)
	Mycosis fungoides
	myocardial fibrosis
M & F	mother and father
MFB	metallic foreign body
MFD	midforceps delivery (obstetrics)
mfd.	microfarad (electrical measurement)
MFT	muscle function test (procedure/physical medicine)
MG	myasthenia gravis
Mg.	magnesium
mg.	milligram
mg%	milligrams percent
	milligrams per hundred milliliters
MGN	membranous glomerulonephritis
$MgSO_4$	magnesium sulfate (medication orders/prescriptions)
MH	marital history
	medical history
	menstrual history
	mental health
MHA	microangiopathic hemolytic anemia
MHB	maximum hospital benefit
MHb	methemoglobin (laboratory/chemistry)
M/hct.	microhematocrit (laboratory/hematology)
MHR	maximum heart rate (during stress test)

MI	mitral insufficiency (incompetence)
	myocardial infarction
MIC	Maternal and Infant Care
	medical intensive care
	minimum inhibitory concentration
micro.	microscopic (microscopy)
	microscopic findings (in urinary sediment)
MICU	medical intensive care unit
	mobile intensive care unit
mid.	middle
mid. sag.	midsagittal
MIFR	maximal inspiratory flow rate (pulmonary function test)
millisec.	millisecond
min.	minimal (minimum)
	minor
	minute
MIP	maximum inspiratory pressure (pulmonary function test)
misc.	miscellaneous
mist.	a mixture (Latin: *mistura*) (prescriptions)
mit. insuf.	mitral insufficiency
mIU	milli-international unit (1/1000 of international unit)
mixt.	mixture (medication orders/prescriptions)
MJ	marijuana
ML	middle lobe (of lung)
	midline

ml.	milliliter
MLAP	mean left atrial pressure
MLC	mixed lymphocyte culture
MLD	minimal lethal dose
ml/min/m²	milliliters per minute per square meter
M/L ratio	monocyte-lymphocyte ratio (laboratory/hematology)
MM	mucous membrane
mM.	millimol (electrolyte measurement)
mm.	millimeter muscles
mm³	cubic millimeter
MMEF	maximal midexpiratory flow (pulmonary function test)
MMEFR	maximal midexpiratory flow rate (pulmonary function test)
M & M enema	milk and molasses enema (procedure/enema)
MMFR	maximal midexpiratory flow rate (pulmonary function test)
mmHg	millimeters of mercury (blood pressure)
mM/L	millimols per liter
mmm.	millimicron (microscopy)
MMPI	Minnesota Multiphasic Personality Inventory (psychological test)
MN	myoneural
M/N	midnight
M & N	morning and night

Mn.	manganese (laboratory/chemistry)
MNCV	motor nerve conduction velocity (procedure/physical medicine)
MO	mineral oil (medication order) minute output (of heart)
Mo.	molybdenum
mo.	month
mob.	mobile (mobility) mobilization
MOD	maturity onset diabetes
mod.	moderate
MOM	milk of magnesia (medication order)
Mono.	infectious mononucleosis
mono.	monocyte (laboratory/hematology)
MOPP	nitrogen mustard, oncovin, procarbazine and prednisone (cancer chemotherapy)
morph.	morphology (morphological)
mort.	mortality
mos.	months
mOsm.	milliosmol
MP	menstrual period metacarpophalangeal (joint) metatarsophalangeal (joint) multiparous
6-MP	6-mercaptopurine (medication order)

MPA	main pulmonary artery
MPAP	mean pulmonary artery pressure
MPI	maximum point of impulse
	multiphasic personality inventory (psychological test)
MPJ	metacarpophalangeal joint
MPS	mucopolysaccharide
MR	mental retardation (mentally retarded)
	metabolic rate
	mitral regurgitation
mr.	milliroentgen (radiation measurement)
M & R	measure and record
MRAP	mean right atrial pressure
MRD	medical record department
MRF	mitral regurgitant flow
M & R I & O	measure and record intake and output (fluids)
MRVP	mean right ventricular pressure
M.R. × 1 . . .	may repeat one time, . . . (medication order)
MS	mental status
	mitral stenosis
	morphine sulfate (medication order)
	multiple sclerosis
	musculoskeletal
MSAP	mean systemic arterial pressure
MSC	medical social coordinator
msec.	millisecond

MSER	mean systolic ejection rate
MSH	melanocyte stimulating hormone
MSL	midsternal line
MST	mean survival time
MSU	mid-stream urine specimen (procedure/urine culture)
MSUD	maple syrup urine disease
MT	empty malignant teratoma maximal therapy metatarsal (joint)
MTC	maximum toxic concentration
MTD	maximum tolerated dose
MTI	minimum time interval
MTP	metatarsophalangeal (joint)
MTU	methylthiouracil
M tuberc.	Mycobacterium tuberculosis
MTX	methotrexate (cancer chemotherapy)
MU	mouse unit (with reference to gonadotropins)
mu (μ)	micron (microscopy measurement)
MUC	mucosal ulcerative colitis
multip.	multiparous
multivits	multivitamins (medication orders/prescriptions)
musc.	muscles (muscular)
MV	minute volume mitral valve mixed venous (blood)

MVR	mitral valve replacement (operation/cardiac)
MVV	maximum voluntary ventilation (pulmonary function test)
My.	myopia (eye examination)
Myco.	Mycobacterium (on bacteriology reports)
myelo.	myelocyte (laboratory/hematology)
MZ	monozygotic

N

N	Negro
	nerve
	neutrophil (on white blood count reports)
	nitrogen
	none
	normal
	number
NA	noradrenaline
	not applicable
	not available
	nurse assistant
	nurse's aide
Na	sodium (laboratory/chemistry)
NaCl	sodium chloride (intravenous solution)

NAD	no acute distress
	no appreciable disease
	normal axis deviation
	nothing abnormal detected
NAG	narrow angle glaucoma
narc.	narcotic (medication order)
NAS	no added salt (diet order)
nas.	nasal
nat.	natural
NB	newborn
	note well (Latin: *nota bene*)
nbl.	normoblast (on hematology reports)
NBM	nothing by mouth (diet order)
NBS	no bacteria seen (microscopy)
NBTE	nonbacterial thrombotic endocarditis
NBW	normal birth weight
NC	neurologic check
	no change
	noncontributory
N/C	no charge
	no complaints
nc.	nanocurie (radioactivity measurement)
NCA	neurocirculatory asthenia
NCC	nursing clerical coordinator

ND	neonatal death
	neurotic depression (psychiatry)
	no data
	no disease
	nondisabling
	normal delivery (obstetrics)
	not detectable
	not detected
	not determined
	not done
N/D	no defects
N_d	refractive index (eye examination)
NDV	Newcastle disease virus
NE	Neomycin (on culture and sensitivity reports)
	nerve excitability
	neurologic examination
	no effect
	norepinephrine
	not enlarged
	not evaluated
	not examined
NED	no evidence of disease
NEEP	negative end-expiratory pressure (respiratory therapy)
NEFA	nonesterified fatty acids (laboratory/chemistry)
neg.	negative
nerv.	nervous
Neuro.	neurology
Neuro-Surg.	neurosurgery
neut.	neutrophil (laboratory/hematology)

NF	Nafcillin (on culture and sensitivity reports)
	National Formulary (drugs)
	Negro female
	not found
NFTD	normal full term delivery
NG	nasogastric (tube)
	nitroglycerin (medication order)
N/G	no good
ng.	nanogram (same as millimicrogram)
NGU	nongonococcal urethritis
NH	nursing home
NH_3	ammonia
NH_4Cl	ammonium chloride (medication orders/prescriptions)
NHS	normal human serum
NI	not identified
	not isolated
NIA	no information available
nil	none
nitro	nitroglycerin (medication order)
n/k	not known
NKHA	nonketotic hyperosmolar acidosis
n/l	normal limits
NM	Negro male
	neuromuscular
	nitrogen mustard (cancer chemotherapy)
	nuclear medicine

n/m	not measured (not measurable)
	not mentioned
NMA	neurogenic muscular atrophy
NMI	no middle initial
NND	neonatal death
n/o	none obtained
no.	number
noc.	night (Latin: *noctis*)
noct.	at night (Latin: *nocte*)
	nocturnal
non rep.	do not repeat (Latin: *non repetatur*) (prescriptions)
	no refill (prescriptions)
non segs.	nonsegmented neutrophils
norm.	normal
NOS	not otherwise specified
NP	nasopharyngeal (nasopharynx)
	neuropathology
	neuropsychiatric
	new patient
	nucleoprotein
	nursing procedure
NPA	near point of accommodation (eye examination)
NPB	nodal premature beat
NPC	near point of convergence (eye examination)
NP cult.	nasopharyngeal culture (procedure/bacteriology)
NPD	Neimann-Pick disease

NPH	neutral protamine Hagedorn (insulin) (medication order) normal pressure hydrocephalus
NPI	no present illness
NPN	nonprotein nitrogen (laboratory/chemistry)
NPO	nothing by mouth (Latin: *non per os*) (diet order)
NR	do not repeat (Latin: *non repetatur*) (prescriptions) nonreactive nonrebreathing (oxygen mask) no refill (prescriptions) no response normal range not readable not recorded
N/R	not remarkable
nr.	near
Nrbc	nucleated red blood cells (on hematology reports)
NRC	normal retinal correspondence (eye examination) not routine care
NREM	nonrapid eye movement
NRI	neutral regular insulin

NS	nephrotic syndrome
	nervous system
	neurosurgery
	nonspecific
	nonsymptomatic
	normal saline
	(intravenous solution)
	normal serum
	no specimen (no sample)
	not significant
	not sufficient (on laboratory reports)
N/S	normal saline
	(intravenous solution)
NSA	no serious (significant) abnormality
NSC	no significant change
NSD	normal spontaneous delivery
	no significant defect
	no significant deviation
	no significant difference
	no significant disease
NSFTD	normal spontaneous full term
	delivery
nsg.	nursing
NSO	Neosporin ointment
	Nursing Service Office
NSQ	not sufficient quantity (on laboratory
	reports)
NSR	normal sinus rhythm (heart)
NSS	normal saline solution
	(intravenous solution)
NSU	nonspecific urethritis
N Surg.	neurosurgery
NT	nasotracheal (tube)
	not tested

N & T	nose and throat
NTG	nitroglycerin (medication order)
	nontoxic goiter
NTN	nephrotoxic nephritis
NTP	nitroprusside
nuc.	nucleated
nucl.	nucleus
NV	normal value (on laboratory reports)
Nv	naked vision (eye examination)
N & V	nausea and vomiting
NVA	near visual acuity (eye examination)
NVD	nausea, vomiting, diarrhea
	neck vein distention
NVS	neurological vital signs
NWB	nonweight bearing
NYD	not yet diagnosed
NYHA	New York Heart Association (classification of heart disease)

O

O	eye (Latin: *oculus*)
	none
	objective (in problem-oriented medical records)
	occiput
	opium
	oral
O₂	oxygen

O2	both eyes (eye examination)
ō	none
o–	ortho (in chemical formulas)
OA	occiput anterior (fetal position)
	old age
	osteoarthritis
O & A	observation and assessment
OAD	obstructive airway disease
OAG	open angle glaucoma
OAP	ophthalmic artery pressure (procedure/ophthalmology)
OB	obstetrics
	occult blood
OBG	obstetrics and gynecology
OB-Gyn.	obstetrics-gynecology
obl.	oblique
OBS	obstetrics
	organic brain syndrome
obs.	observed (observation)
obst.	obstetrics
	obstruction
OC	on call
	oral contraceptive
O & C	onset and course
O_2 cap.	oxygen capacity (laboratory/blood gas)
occ.	occasionally
	occurrence
occup.	occupation (occupational)
OCT	ornithine carbamyl transferase (laboratory/chemistry)

OCV	ordinary conversational voice
OD	on duty
	open drop (ether anesthesia)
	optical density
	outside diameter
	overdose (drugs)
	right eye (Latin: *oculus dexter*)
o.d.	daily
	(medication orders/prescriptions)
	every day
	(medication orders/prescriptions)
	once daily (Latin: *omni die*)
	(medication orders/prescriptions)
ODA	right occiput anterior (fetal position)
ODM	ophthalmodynamometry
	(procedure/ophthalmology)
ODP	right occiput posterior (fetal position)
ODT	right occiput transverse (fetal position)
OFC	occipital-frontal circumference (head)
off.	office
	official
OGTT	oral glucose tolerance test
	(diabetes detection)
	(laboratory/chemistry)
OH	occupational history
	open heart (surgery)
17-OH	17-hydroxycorticosteroids (17-OHCS)
	(laboratory/endocrinology)
OHCS	hydroxycorticosteroid
OHD	organic heart disease
OIH	ovulation-inducing hormone

oint.	ointment (medication orders/prescriptions)
o.j.	orange juice (diet order)
OK	all right approved correct
ol.	oil (prescriptions)
ol. oliv.	olive oil (Latin: *oleum olivea*)
OM	otitis media
o.m.	every morning (Latin: *omni mane*) (medication orders/prescriptions)
OMI	old myocardial infarction
OMPA	otitis media, purulent, acute
OMSA	otitis media, suppurative, acute
OMSC	otitis media, suppurative, chronic
OMVC	open mitral valve commissurotomy (operation/heart)
OOB	out of bed
OP	old (previously seen) patient opening pressure operative procedure osmotic pressure outpatient
op.	operation
O & P	ova and parasites (laboratory/bacteriology)
OPB	outpatient basis
OPD	outpatient department
oper.	operation

Ophth.	ophthalmology
opp.	opposite
OPS	outpatient service
OPT	outpatient treatment
opt.	optimum optional
OR	operating room
OR enema	oil retention enema (procedure/enema)
org.	organic
ORIF	open reduction with internal fixation (operation/orthopedics)
orig.	origin (originated) original
ORL	otorhinolaryngology
Ortho.	orthopedics
OS	left eye (Latin: *oculus sinister*) opening snap (heart sound) oral surgery
O$_2$ sat.	oxygen saturation (laboratory/blood gas)
osm.	osmotic
osmo.	osmolality (on laboratory reports)
osteo.	osteoarthritis osteomyelitis
OT	occupational therapy ocular tension (eye examination) orotracheal (tube)

OTC	over-the-counter (drugs)
	oxytetracycline (on culture and sensitivity reports)
OTD	organ tolerance dose
Oto.	otolaryngology
	otology
OU	both eyes together (Latin: *oculi unitas*)
	observation unit
OURQ	outer upper right quadrant (breast)
OV	office visit
O/W	oil in water (medication base)
oz.	ounce

P

P	parent
	parity (obstetrics)
	partial pressure (blood gases)
	Pasteurella (on bacteriology reports)
	penicillin (on culture and sensitivity reports)
	percussion
	phosphorus (laboratory/chemistry)
	plan (on problem-oriented medical records)
	plasma
	posterior
	pressure
	private (patient or room)
	protein (on diet orders)
	pulse
	pupil

^{32}P	radioactive phosphorus (nuclear medicine)
P_1	first parental generation
P_2	second pulmonic heart sound
$\bar{p}$	after (Latin: *post*) following
p–	para (in chemical formulas)
PA	paralysis agitans pernicious anemia physician's assistant posterior-anterior (chest x-ray) primary anemia prolonged action (tablets) pulmonary artery
P & A	percussion and auscultation
$P(A\text{-}aDO_2)$	alveolar-arterial oxygen tension difference (pulmonary function test)
PABA	para-aminobenzoic acid (medication order)
PAC	phenacetin, aspirin, caffeine (medication orders/prescriptions) premature atrial contraction
$PaCO_2$	arterial carbon dioxide tension (laboratory/blood gas)
PAH	para-aminohippuric acid (kidney function test) pulmonary artery hypertension
PAL	posterior axillary line
palp.	palpable (palpate)
palpit.	palpitations
PAN	polyarteritis nodosa

panendo.	panendoscopy (procedure/gastroenterology)
PaO_2	arterial oxygen pressure tension (laboratory/blood gas)
PAP	primary atypical pneumonia pulmonary alveolar proteinosis pulmonary artery pressure
Pap.	Papanicolaou smear (procedure/gynecology)
PAR	perennial allergic rhinitis
para.	paraplegic
Para I, Para II, . . .	having borne one child, two children, . . .
paracent.	paracentesis (procedure/surgery)
par. aff.	to the part affected (Latin: *pars affecta*) (medication orders/prescriptions)
parent.	parenteral (parenterally)
parox.	paroxysmal
part aeq.	in equal parts (Latin: *partes aequales*) (prescriptions)
PARU	postanesthetic recovery unit
PAS	para-aminosalicylic acid (medication order) periodic-acid-Schiff (stain) pulmonary artery stenosis
pass.	passive
Past.	Pasteurella (on bacteriology reports)
PAT	paroxysmal atrial tachycardia

Path.	pathology
pat. med.	patent medicine
PA-VF	pulmonary arteriovenous fistula
PAWP	pulmonary artery wedge pressure
PB	Polymyxin B (on culture and sensitivity reports)
Pb	lead (Latin: *plumbum*) presbyopia (eye examination)
pb.	phenobarbital
P & B	phenobarbital and belladonna
PBC	primary biliary cirrhosis
PBF	pulmonary blood flow
PBG	porphobilinogen (laboratory/chemistry)
PBI	protein-bound iodine (laboratory/endocrinology)
pbo.	placebo
PBV	predicted blood volume
PBZ	Pyribenzamine
PC	phosphocreatine platelet count portacaval (shunt) present complaint Professional Corporation (physician)
p.c.	after food (Latin: *post cibum*) (diet order)
PCB	paracervical block (procedure/anesthesiology)
PcB	near point of convergence to the base line (eye examination)
PCc	periscopic concave (eye examination)

PCD	polycystic disease
PCF	prothrombin conversion factor
PCG	phonocardiogram (procedure/cardiology)
PCH	paroxysmal cold hemoglobinuria
PCN	penicillin (medication order)
pCO_2	partial pressure of carbon dioxide (laboratory/blood gas)
PCS	portacaval shunt (operation/liver) postcardiotomy syndrome
PCT	porphyria cutanea tarda proximal convoluted tubule (kidney)
PCU	protective care unit
PCV	packed cell volume (laboratory/hematology)
PCW pressure	pulmonary capillary wedge pressure
PCx	periscopic convex (eye examination)
PD	Parkinson's disease poorly differentiated (cells) pregnanediol progression of disease pulmonary disease
p/d	packs per day (cigarettes)
PDA	patent ductus arteriosus
PDR	Physician's Desk Reference (book)
pdr.	powder (medication orders/prescriptions)
PE	pharyngoesophageal physical examination

	pleural effusion
	pulmonary edema
	pulmonary embolism
P_E	expiratory pressure (respiratory therapy)
PEARLA	pupils equal and react to light and accommodation
Ped.	pediatrics
PEEP	positive end expiratory pressure (respiratory therapy)
PEF	peak expiratory flow (pulmonary function test)
PEFR	peak expiratory flow rate (pulmonary function test)
PEG	pneumoencephalogram (procedure/neurology)
Pen.	penicillin (medication order)
pent.	pentothal (anesthetic agent)
PEP	pre-ejection period (heart)
per	by for each
per.	period (periodic)
perf.	perforation (perforated) performed
periap.	periapical
PERLA	pupils equal, react to light and accommodation
perm.	permanent
PERRLA	pupils equal, round, react to light and accommodation

pers.	personal
PET	pre-eclamptic toxemia
PETN	pentaerythrityl tetranitrate
PFO	patent foramen ovale
PFR	peak flow rate (pulmonary function test)
PFT	pulmonary function test
PG	paregoric prostaglandin pyoderma gangrenosum
Pg.	pregnant
pg.	picogram (same as micromicrogram)
PGH	pituitary growth hormone
PH	past history personal history prostatic hypertrophy public health pulmonary hypertension
Ph[1]	Philadelphia chromosome (laboratory/hematology)
PHA	phytohemagglutinin (laboratory/serology)
phar.	pharmacy
pheno.	phenotype
PHN	public health nurse
phos.	phosphate phosphorus (laboratory/chemistry)
PHP	pseudohypoparathyroidism
phys.	physical physician

phys. dis.	physical disability
Phys. Med.	physical medicine
PI	peripheral iridectomy (operation/ophthalmology) present illness pulmonary infarction
P_I	inspiratory pressure (respiratory therapy)
PIA	plasma insulin activity (laboratory/endocrinology)
PICU	pediatric intensive care unit pulmonary intensive care unit
PID	pelvic inflammatory disease prolapsed intervertebral disc
PIE	pulmonary infiltration with eosinophilia
PIFR	peak inspiratory flow rate (respiratory therapy)
pil	pills (medication orders/prescriptions)
PIPJ	proximal interphalangeal joint
PIVD	protruded intervertebral disc
PJB	premature junctional beat (ECG)
PJT	paroxysmal junctional tachycardia
PK	Prausnitz-Küstner (reaction) pyruvate kinase assay (laboratory/chemistry)
PKU	phenylketonuria
PL	perception of light (eye examination)
pl.	place plasma (on laboratory reports)

plat.	platelets (laboratory/hematology)
PM	after death (Latin: *post mortem*)
	after noon (Latin: *post meridian*)
	night
	petit mal (seizures)
	physical medicine
	polymorphs (white blood cells)
	presystolic murmur
PMA	progressive muscular atrophy
PMB	post menopausal bleeding
PMD	primary myocardial disease
	progressive muscular dystrophy
PMH	past medical history
PMI	past medical illness
	point of maximum impulse
	point of maximum intensity
	previous medical illness
PMN's	polymorphonucleocytes
PMP	past menstrual period
PMR	physical medicine and rehabilitation
PMS	post menopausal syndrome
PMT	premenstrual tension
PN	peripheral nerve
	peripheral neuropathy
Pn.	pneumonia
P & N	psychiatry and neurology
PNC	premature nodal contraction
PND	paroxysmal nocturnal dyspnea
	postnasal drip
pneumo.	pneumothorax

PNH	paroxysmal nocturnal hemoglobinuria
PNS	parasympathetic nervous system peripheral nervous system
pnx.	pneumothorax
PO	postoperative
P/O	phone order
P_O	opening pressure
p.o.	by mouth (Latin: *per os*)
PO_2	partial pressure of oxygen (laboratory/blood gas)
PO_4	phosphate
POA	primary optic atrophy
POC	postoperative care
POD	postoperative day
PODx.	preoperative diagnosis
poik.	poikilocytosis (of blood cells)
polio	poliomyelitis
polys	polymorphonuclear leukocytes (laboratory/hematology)
POMP	prednisone, oncovin, methotrexate and 6-mercaptopurine (cancer chemotherapy)
POMR	problem-oriented medical record
poplit.	popliteal
pos.	position positive
pos. press.	positive pressure
poss.	possible

post.	posterior
	post mortem (autopsy)
postop.	postoperative
pot.	potassium (laboratory/chemistry)
powd.	powder
PP	postpartum
	postprandial
	private patient
	prothrombin-proconvertin
	proximal phalanx
	pulse pressure
pp	near point of accommodation (eye examination)
PPA	palpitation, percussion, auscultation
PPBS	postprandial blood sugar (laboratory/chemistry)
PPC	progressive patient care
PPD	purified protein derivative (procedure/tuberculin skin test)
PPF	plasma protein fraction
PPH	postpartum hemorrhage
	primary pulmonary hypertension
PPHP	pseudo-pseudohypoparathyroidism
PPLO	pleuropneumonia-like organism
ppm	parts per million
ppt.	precipitate
pptd.	precipitated
PPV	positive pressure ventilation (respiratory therapy)

PR	Panama red (variation of marijuana)
	partial remission
	peer review
	peripheral resistance
	pulse rate
Pr.	presbyopia (eye examination)
pr.	pair
p.r.	per rectum
P & R	pelvic and rectal (examination)
	pulse and respiration
PRA	plasma renin activity (laboratory/endocrinology)
prac.	practice
pract.	practical
PRBC	packed red blood cells (blood transfusion)
PRC	plasma renin concentration
PRD	postradiation dysplasia
PRE	progressive resistive exercises (physical therapy)
pref.	preference
preg.	pregnant
pregang.	preganglionic
prelim.	preliminary
premie	premature infant
prenat.	prenatal
preop.	preoperative
prep.	prepare (preparation)
press.	pressure

prev.	prevent (prevention)
	previous
PRF	prolactin releasing factor
primip.	woman bearing first child
princ.	principal
	principle
priv.	private
	privilege
PRL	prolactin
p.r.n.	as required
	whenever necessary
	(Latin: *pro re nata*)
	(medication order)
prob.	probable
proc.	procedure
	proceeding
	process
Proct.	proctology
procto.	proctoscopy
	(procedure/rectal)
prod.	product
prof.	profession
prog.	prognosis
	progress
proj.	project
PROM	premature rupture of membranes
pron.	pronation
proph.	prophylactic
prost.	prostate
prosth.	prosthesis

Prot.	Protestant
prot.	protein
prothr. cont.	prothrombin content (laboratory/coagulation)
pro. time	prothrombin time (laboratory/coagulation)
Pro-X	prothrombin time (laboratory/coagulation)
prox.	proximal
PRP	platelet-rich plasma (transfusion)
PS	periodic syndrome physical status plastic surgery pulmonary stenosis pyloric stenosis
P & S	paracentesis and suction (procedure/gastrointestinal)
PSC	posterior subcapsular cataract
PSE	portal systemic encephalopathy
PSG	presystolic gallop
PSGN	poststreptococcal glomerulonephritis
psi	pounds per square inch (pressure measurement)
PSMA	progressive spinal muscular atrophy
PSP	phenolsuflonphthalein (kidney function test)
PSRO	Professional Standard Review Organization
PSS	physiological saline solution (intravenous solution)

P. Surg.	plastic surgery
PSVT	paroxysmal superventricular tachycardia
Psych.	psychiatry
	psychology
PT	parathyroid
	paroxysmal tachycardia
	physical therapy
	physical training
	posterior tibial (pulse)
	prothrombin time (laboratory/coagulation)
P & T	permanent and total (disability)
Pt.	platinum
pt.	part
	patient
	pint
	point
PTA	plasma thromboplastin antecedent (Factor X) (laboratory/coagulation)
	prior to admission (arrival)
	prothrombin activity
p'tase	phosphatase (laboratory/chemistry)
PTC	plasma thromboplastin component (Factor IX) (laboratory/coagulation)
PTE	parathyroid extract
PTED	pulmonary thromboembolic disease
PTH	parathyroid hormone
PTMDF	pupils, tension, media, disc, fundus

P_{Tr}	inspiratory triggering pressure (respiratory therapy)
PTT	partial thromboplastin time (laboratory/coagulation)
PTU	propylthiouracil
PU	pass urine peptic ulcer
PUC	pediatric urine collector
PUD	pulmonary disease
PUE	pyrexia (fever) of unknown etiology
PUFA	polyunsaturated fatty acid
pulm.	pulmonary
pulv.	powder (medication orders/prescriptions)
PUO	pyrexia (fever) of unknown origin
PV	peripheral vascular peripheral vein plasma volume polycythemia vera portal vein
P & V	pyloroplasty and vagotomy (operation/stomach)
PVA	polyvinyl alcohol
PVB	premature ventricular beat
PVC	polyvinyl chloride premature ventricular contraction pulmonary venous congestion
PVD	peripheral vascular disease posterior vitreous detachment (eye) pulmonary vascular disease
PVF	portal venous flow

PvO$_2$	partial pressure of venous oxygen (laboratory/blood gas)
PVP	peripheral venous pressure portal venous pressure
PVR	peripheral vascular resistance pulmonary vascular resistance
PVT	paroxysmal ventricular tachycardia
pvt.	private
PW	posterior wall
PWB	partial weight-bearing
PWC	physical work capacity
PX	physical examination
Px.	prognosis
PZA	pyrazinamide (antitubercular drug)
PZI	protamine zinc insulin (medication order)

Q

Q	quantity volume of blood flow
$\dot{Q}$	rate of blood flow
q.	each every (Latin: *quaque*)
q.a.m.	every morning
q.d.	every day (Latin: *quaque die*)
q. 2 d.	every second day
q.h.	every hour
q. 2 h.	every two hours

q.i.d.	four times a day (Latin: *quater in die*)
qns	quantity not sufficient (on laboratory reports)
QO$_2$	oxygen consumption (pulmonary function test)
q.o.d.	every other day
q.o.h.	every other hour
q.o.n.	every other night
q.s.	as much as will suffice (Latin: *quantum sufficit*) sufficient quantity (Latin: *quantum satis*) (prescriptions)
q.s. ad	to a sufficient quantity (prescriptions)
qt.	quart
quad.	quadriplegic
qual.	qualitative
quant.	quantitative quantity
q.v.	as much as you wish (Latin: *quantum vis*)

R

R	rate respirations rhythm right
Ⓡ	right

r	roentgen (x-ray measurement)
R−	Rinne's test negative (hearing test)
R+	Rinne's test positive (hearing test)
(R)	rectal (on temperature records)
RA	renal artery repeat action rheumatoid agglutinins (laboratory/serology) rheumatoid arthritis right arm right atrial (atrium)
R_A	airway resistance (pulmonary function test)
Ra	radium (nuclear medicine)
RAD	right axis deviation (ECG)
rad.	radial radical radius
Radiol.	radiology
RAE	right atrial enlargement
RA factor	rheumatoid arthritis factor (laboratory/serology)
RAH	right atrial hypertrophy
RAI	radioactive iodine (nuclear medicine)
RAIU	radioactive iodine uptake (nuclear medicine)
RALT	routine admission laboratory tests
RAO	right anterior oblique
RAP	right atrial pressure

RAT	right anterior thigh (injection site)
RB	right buttock (injection site)
RBBB	right bundle branch block (ECG)
RBC	red blood count (laboratory/hematology)
r.b.c.	red blood cells
RBCV	red blood cell volume (laboratory/hematology)
RBD	right border of dullness
RBF	renal blood flow
RCA	right coronary artery
RCD	relative area of cardiac dullness
RCM	right costal margin
RCS	reticulum cell sarcoma
RCU	respiratory care unit
RCV	red cell volume (laboratory/hematology)
RD	Raynaud's disease
	respiratory disease
	retinal detachment
	right deltoid (injection site)
RDDA	recommended daily dietary allowance
RDI	rupture delivery interval (obstetrics)
RDS	respiratory distress syndrome
RDT	regular dialysis treatment
RE	regional enteritis
	reticulo-endothelium
rec.	record

RECG	radioelectrocardiology (telemetry) (procedure/cardiology)
recip.	recipient
recond.	reconditioning
reconstr.	reconstruction
rect.	rectum (rectal)
recur.	recurrent (recurrence)
ref.	refer reference
ref. doc.	referring doctor
ref. phys.	referring physician
reg.	region regular
regen.	regenerate (regeneration)
rehab.	rehabilitation
rel.	relation relative
REM	rapid eye movement
rem.	remove
rep.	let it be repeated (Latin: *repetatur*) (prescriptions) report
RES	reticuloendothelial system
res.	research reserve residence resident
resp.	respectively respiration respiratory responsible

ret.	retired
ret. cath.	retention catheter
retic. ct.	reticulocyte count (laboratory/hematology)
retics	reticulocytes (laboratory/hematology)
rev.	review revision
RF	respiratory failure rheumatic fever rheumatoid factor
RFA	right femoral artery
RFB	retained foreign body
RFS	renal function studies
RG	right gluteus (injection site)
RH	reactive hyperemia right hand
Rh+	Rhesus positive (blood) (laboratory/blood bank)
Rh−	Rhesus negative (blood) (laboratory/blood bank)
Rh agglut.	rheumatoid agglutinins (laboratory/serology)
RHC	respirations have ceased
RHD	relative hepatic dullness renal hypertensive disease rheumatic heart disease
rheum.	rheumatic
RHF	right heart failure
Rh factor	Rhesus factor (laboratory/blood bank)

Rhin.	rhinology
RHL	right hepatic lobe
rhm	roentgen (per) hour (at one) meter (radiation therapy)
RI	refractive index (eye examination) regional ileitis respiratory illness
RIA	radioimmunoassay (laboratory method)
RICU	respiratory intensive care unit
RIF	right iliac fossa (injection site)
RISA	radioactive iodine serum albumin (nuclear medicine)
RIU	radioactive iodine uptake (nuclear medicine)
RK	right kidney
RL	right leg right lung
R→L	right to left
RLC	residual lung capacity (pulmonary function test)
RLD	related living donor
RLE	right lower extremity
RLF	retrolental fibroplasia
RLL	right lower lobe (lung)
RLQ	right lower quadrant
RLR	right lateral rectus
RLS	Ringer's lactate solution (intravenous solution)
RLT	right lateral thigh (injection site)

RM	radical mastectomy (operation/breast)
	respiratory movement
	ruptured membranes (obstetrics)
RML	right mediolateral (episiotomy) (operation/obstetrics)
	right middle lobe (lung)
RMR	right medial rectus (eye examination)
RMSF	Rocky Mountain spotted fever
RMV	respiratory minute volume (pulmonary function test)
RN	Registered Nurse
Rn	radon (radiation measurement)
RNA	ribonucleic acid
RNase	ribonuclease
RND	radical neck dissection (operation/neck)
RO	routine order
R/O	rule out
ROA	right occiput anterior (fetal position)
Roent.	roentgenology (x-ray)
ROM	range-of-motion
	rupture of membranes (obstetrics)
ROP	right occiput posterior (fetal position)
ROS	review of systems
ROT	remedial occupational therapy
	right occiput transverse (fetal position)
rot.	rotate (rotating)

rout.	routine
R_p	pulmonary resistance (pulmonary function test)
RPA	right pulmonary artery
RPF	Reiter protein complement fixation test (laboratory/serology) relaxed pelvic floor renal plasma flow
RPG	retrograde pyelogram (x-ray/kidneys)
RPP	retropubicprostatectomy (operation/urology)
RPR	rapid plasma reagin (test) (laboratory/serology)
RPV	right pulmonary vein
RQ	respiratory quotient
RR	radiation response recovery room respiratory rate
R & R	rate and rhythm (heart)
RRE	round, regular, equal (eye examination)
rRNA	ribosomal ribonucleic acid
RRP	relative refractory period (heart)
RS	rectal suppository (prescriptions) review of symptoms rhythm strip (electrocardiogram) right side Ringer's solution (intravenous solution)

RSB	right sternal border
RSIVP	rapid sequence intravenous pyelogram (x-ray/kidneys)
RSO	right salpingo-oophorectomy (operation/gynecology)
RSR	regular sinus rhythm (heart)
RSV	right subclavian vein
RT	respiratory therapist respiratory therapy
rt.	right
RTA	renal tubular acidosis
RTC	return to clinic
rtd.	retarded
rt. lat.	right lateral
RTN	renal tubular necrosis
RT$_3$U	resin triiodothyronine uptake (laboratory/endocrinology)
RU	right upper roentgen unit (radiation therapy)
RUE	right upper extremity
RUL	right upper lobe (lung)
rupt.	rupture
RUQ	right upper quadrant
RUR	resin uptake ratio (nuclear medicine)
RV	residual volume (pulmonary function test) right ventricle
RVD	relative vertebral density

RVE	right ventricular enlargement
RVEDP	right ventricular end diastolic pressure
RVH	right ventricular hypertrophy
RVO	relaxed vaginal outlet
RVRC	renal vein renin concentration
RVT	renal vein thrombosis
RV/TLC	residual volume per total lung compliance (pulmonary function test)
Rx.	drugs
	medication
	prescription
	take (Latin: *recipe*)
	therapy
	treatment

S

S	sacral (vertebrae)
	saline
	section
	single (marital status)
	son
	streptomycin (on culture and sensitivity reports)
s	sign
S_1	first heart sound
S_2	second heart sound
S_3	third heart sound
S_4	fourth heart sound

S1, S2, . . .	first sacral vertebra, second sacral vertebra, . . .
s̄	without (Latin: *sine*)
SA	serum albumin sinoatrial (node) Stokes-Adams (attacks) surface area sustained action (drugs)
S/A	sugar and acetone (laboratory/urinalysis)
SAH	subarachnoid hemorrhage
Sal.	salmonella (on bacteriology reports)
sal.	salicylate saline
sanit.	sanitarium sanitary
SAP	serum alkaline phosphatase (laboratory/chemistry) systemic arterial pressure
SAS	supravalvular aortic stenosis
sat.	saturate (saturated)
sat. sol.	saturated solution (prescriptions)
SB	serum bilirubin single breath small bowel Stanford-Binet (intelligence test) sternal border stillborn
Sb.	strabismus (eye examination)
SBC	special back care strict bed confinement

SBE	subacute bacterial endocarditis
SBP	systolic blood pressure
SBR	strict bed rest
SC	sickle cell (anemia) special care sternoclavicular (joint)
sc.	subcutaneous (injection site) without correction (eye examination)
SCABG	single coronary artery bypass graft (operation/heart)
SCC	squamous cell carcinoma
S-C disease	sickle cell-hemoglobin C disease
sched.	schedule
schiz.	schizophrenia
SCK	serum creatine kinase (laboratory/chemistry)
sclero.	scleroderma
scop.	scopolamine (medication order)
SD	septal defect (heart) spontaneous delivery sudden death
SDS	sensory deprivation syndrome
sds.	sounds
SE	saline enema (procedure/enema) status epilepticus
^{75}Se	radioactive selenomethionine (nuclear medicine)
sec.	second secondary

sect.	section
SED	skin erythema dose
sed. rate	sedimentation rate (laboratory/hematology)
segs.	segmented white cells (on white blood count reports)
SEM	systolic ejection murmur
sem. ves.	seminal vesicles
sens.	sensitivity (on culture reports)
SEP	systolic ejection period
sep.	separate (separately)
sept.	septum
seq.	sequence sequestrum
serv.	service
sev.	several severe severed
SE valve	Starr-Edwards (heart) valve
SF	scarlet fever spinal fluid streptococcus faecalis (on bacteriology reports)
SFA	superficial femoral artery
SFP	spinal fluid pressure
SFS	serial focal seizures
SFT	skinfold thickness
SG	skin graft (plastic surgery) specific gravity (urine)

SGOT	serum glutamic oxaloacetic transaminase (laboratory/chemistry)
SGPT	serum glutamic pyruvic transaminase (laboratory/chemistry)
SH	serum hepatitis social history somatotrophic (growth) hormone
sh.	short shoulder
S & H	speech and hearing
Shig.	Shigella (laboratory/bacteriology)
SHO	secondary hypertrophic osteoarthropathy
SI	serum iron
Si	silicon
sib.	sibling
SICU	surgical intensive care unit
SIDS	sudden infant death syndrome
sig.	let it be labeled (Latin: *signetur*) (prescriptions) significant
sigmo.	sigmoidoscopy (procedure/intestinal)
SIW	self-inflicted wound
SK	streptokinase (on culture and sensitivity reports)
SL	slit lamp (eye examination) streptolysin sublingual (medication orders/prescriptions)

sl.	slight (slightly)
	slow
SLB	short leg brace
SLDH	serum lactic dehydrogenase (laboratory/chemistry)
SLE	systemic lupus erythematosus
SLEV	St. Louis encephalitis virus
SLO	streptolysin-O
SLR	straight leg raising
sl. tr.	slight trace (on laboratory reports)
SM	simple mastectomy
	streptomycin (on culture and sensitivity reports)
	systolic mean (pressure)
	systolic murmur
sm.	small
SMA-6	Sequential Multiple Analysis-6 tests (laboratory/chemistry)
SMA-12	Sequential Multiple Analysis-12 tests (laboratory/chemistry)
sm. amts.	small amounts
SMBFT	small bowel follow-through (x-ray/intestinal)
SMC	special mouth care
SMR	skeletal muscle relaxant (drug)
	submucous resection (operation/nose)
SMS	serial motor seizures
SMX	sulfamethoxazole (on culture and sensitivity reports)

SN	standard nomenclature (records) student nurse suprasternal notch
SNB	scalene node biopsy (operation/chest)
SNS	sympathetic nervous system
SO	salpingo-oophorectomy (operation/gynecology)
SO_4	sulphate
SOAA	signed out against advice
SOAP	subjective, objective, assessment plan (in problem-oriented medical records)
SOB	short of breath
sol.	solution (prescriptions)
solv.	dissolve (Latin: *solve*) (prescriptions) solvent
SOM	serious otitis media superior oblique muscle (eye)
SOMA	signed out against medical advice
SONP	solid organs not palpable
SOP	standard operating procedure
s.o.s.	one dose if necessary (Latin: *si opus sit*) (medication order)
SP	systolic pressure
sp.	space specific spinal

S/P	semi-private (room)
	status post (no change–as before)
SPA	salt poor albumin
	(intravenous therapy)
spans.	spansules
	(prescriptions)
SPCA	serum prothrombin conversion
	accelerator (Factor VII)
sp. cd.	spinal cord
spec.	special
	specific
	specimen (laboratory)
SPEP	serum protein electrophoresis
	(laboratory/chemistry)
sp. fl.	spinal fluid
sp. gr.	specific gravity (urine)
sph.	spherical
spont.	spontaneous
SPP	suprapubic prostatectomy
	(operation/urology)
spt.	spirits (alcohol)
SQ	subcutaneous (injection site)
sq.	squamous (cell)
	square
sq. cell ca.	squamous cell carcinoma
sq. epith.	squamous epithelium
SR	sedimentation rate
	sinus rhythm (heart)
	systems review (patient's history)
^{85}SR	radioactive strontium
	(nuclear medicine)

SRM	superior rectus muscle (eye)
SS	saline soak
	saturated solution
	(prescriptions)
	side to side
	Social Security
	social service
	sterile solution
S & S	signs and symptoms
s͞s	one-half (Latin: *semissen*)
	(medication orders/prescriptions)
SSE	soapsuds enema
	(procedure/enema)
SS enema	saline solution enema
	(procedure/enema)
SSKI	saturated solution of potassium
	iodide
	(medication orders/prescriptions)
SSLI	serum sickness-like illness
SSS	sick sinus syndrome
	sterile saline soak
ST	sinus tachycardia
	speech therapist
stand.	standard (standardized)
staph.	staphylococcus
	(laboratory/bacteriology)
stat.	immediately (Latin: *statim*)
stb.	stillborn
STC	soft tissue calcification
STD	skin test dose
std.	standard

stet	let it stand
STF	special tube feeding
STG	split thickness graft (operation/plastic surgery)
STH	somatotrophic (growth) hormone subtotal hysterectomy (operation/gynecology)
stillb.	stillborn
stim.	stimulus (stimulate)
str.	straight
Strab.	strabismus (eye examination)
strep.	streptococcus (laboratory/bacteriology)
struc.	structure (structural)
STS	serological test for syphilis (laboratory/serology) standard test for syphilis (laboratory/serology)
STU	skin test unit
SUA	serum uric acid (laboratory/chemistry)
subcrep.	subcrepitant (rales)
subcut.	subcutaneous (subcutaneously)
subling.	sublingual (under tongue) (medication orders/prescriptions)
submand.	submandibular
SUD	sudden unexpected (unexplained) death
suff.	sufficient
SUID	sudden unexplained infant death

SUN	serum urea nitrogen (laboratory/chemistry)
sup.	superior supination
supp.	suppository (medication orders/prescriptions) suppurative
Surg.	surgery (surgical or surgeon)
susp.	suspension
SV	snake venom stroke volume subclavian vein supraventricular
SVC	selective venous catheterization superior vena cava
SVCG	spatial vectorcardiogram (procedure/cardiology)
SVD	spontaneous vaginal delivery
SVE	supraventricular ectopic (beat)
SVG	saphenous vein graft (operation/coronary bypass)
SVI	stroke volume index
SVR	alcohol, whiskey (Latin: *spiritus vini rectificatus*) systemic vascular resistance
SVT	supraventricular tachycardia
SW	social worker
S & W enema	soap and water enema (procedure/enema)
SWI	stroke work index
Sx.	symptoms

sym.	symmetry (symmetrical)
symb.	symbol
sympat.	sympathetic (nervous system)
sympt.	symptom
syn.	synovial (fluid)
	synovitis
synd.	syndrome
syph.	syphilis
syr.	syrup
	(prescriptions)
sys.	system (systemic)
syst.	systemic
	systolic
Sz.	schizophrenia
	seizure

T

T	tablespoonful
	temperature
	thoracic
	Treponema (on bacteriology reports)
	Trichophyton (on bacteriology reports)
	Trypanosoma (on bacteriology reports)
	tumor
t	teaspoonful
	three times (Latin: *ter*)
	time
T₁	tricuspid first heart sound

T$_2$	tricuspid second heart sound
T1, T2, . . .	first thoracic vertebra, second thoracic vertebra, . . .
T−1, T−2, . . .	stages of decreased intraocular tension (eye examination)
T+1, T+2, . . .	stages of increased intraocular tension (eye examination)
TA	therapeutic abortion (operation/gynecology) toxin-antitoxin
T(A)	temperature, axillary (on temperature charts)
T & A	tonsillectomy and adenoidectomy (operation/nose and throat)
tab.	tablet (medication orders/prescriptions)
TAC	triamcinolone cream
TACE	tripara-anisylchloroethylene (medication order)
TAH	total abdominal hysterectomy (operation/gynecology)
talc	talcum powder
TAO	thromboangitis obliterans
TAT	tetanus antitoxin (medication order) thromboplastin activation test
TB	total base tracheobronchitis tubercle bacillus tuberculosis
TBB	transbronchial biopsy (procedure/thoracic surgery)

tbc.	tuberculosis
TBG	thyroxine-binding globulin
TBI	total body irradiation
TBM	tuberculous meningitis
TBNA	treated but not admitted
TBP	thyroxine-binding protein
tbsp.	tablespoonful
TBV	total blood volume
TBW	total body water total body weight

TC	tetracycline (on culture and
	   sensitivity reports)
	throat culture
	tissue culture
	total capacity (lung)
	   (pulmonary function test)
	tubocurarine (on anesthesia reports)

T & C	turn and cough type and crossmatch (laboratory/blood bank)
^{99m}TC	radioactive technetium (nuclear medicine)
TCA	terminal cancer
TCABG	triple coronary artery bypass graft (operation/heart)
TC & DB	turn, cough and deep breathe
TCI	transient cerebral ischemia
TD	thoracic duct total disability transverse diameter (of heart)
T/D	treatment discontinued

TE	tetracycline (on culture and sensitivity reports) tracheoesophageal
T_E	expiratory phase time (pulmonary function test)
T & E	trial and error
teasp.	teaspoonful
tech.	technical technician
T-E fistula	tracheal esophageal fistula
TEM	triethylenemelamine (cancer chemotherapy)
temp.	temperature temporal temporary
term.	terminal terminate (termination)
tert.	tertiary
tet. tox.	tetanus toxoid (medication order)
TF	tactile fremitus tetralogy of Fallot thymol flocculation (laboratory/chemistry) to follow transfer factor
TFA	total fatty acids (laboratory/chemistry)
TFS	testicular feminization syndrome
TG	thyroglobulin triglycerides (laboratory/chemistry)

TGL	triglyceride lipase triglycerides 　(laboratory/chemistry)
TGT	thromboplastin generation test
TGV	transposition of the great vessels
TH	thyroid hormone (thyroxine) total hysterectomy 　(operation/gynecology)
th.	thoracic (thorax)
Thal.	thalassemia
TH & C	terpin hydrate and codeine 　(medication order)
theor.	theoretical
ther.	therapy
therm.	thermal thermometer
thromb.	thrombosis
thym. turb.	thymol turbidity 　(laboratory/chemistry)
TI	time interval tricuspid insufficiency
T$_I$	inspiratory phase time 　(pulmonary function test)
TIA	transient ischemic attack
TIBC	total iron-binding capacity 　(laboratory/chemistry)
t.i.d.	three times daily 　(Latin: *ter in die*) 　(medication orders/prescriptions)
TIE	transient ischemic episode

tinct.	tincture (prescriptions)
T_3 Index	triiodothyroxine index (laboratory/endocrinology)
T_I/T_E	inspiratory-expiratory phase time ratio (pulmonary function test)
titr.	titrate
TJ	triceps jerk (neurologic examination)
TKO	to keep open (intravenous therapy)
TL	Team Leader total lipids (laboratory/chemistry) tubal ligation (operation/gynecology)
TLC	tender loving care thin layer chromatography total lung capacity (pulmonary function test) total lung compliance (pulmonary function test)
TLV	total lung volume (pulmonary function test)
TM	temporomandibular (joint) transcendental meditation transmetatarsal (foot) tympanic membrane (ear)
Tm	maximum tubular clearance (renal function test)
TMA	transmetatarsal amputation (operation/orthopedics)

TME	transmural enteritis
Tm_G	maximum glucose reabsorptive capacity (renal function test)
TMJ	temporomandibular joint
^{Tm}PAH	maximum tubular excretory capacity for para-aminohippurate (renal function test)
Tn	intraocular tension, normal (eye examination)
TčNM	tumor with node metastasis
TNTC	too numerous to count (on laboratory reports)
T(O)	temperature, oral (on temperature records)
T/O	telephone order
TOA	tubo-ovarian abscess
tol.	tolerate (tolerated)
top.	topical (topically) (medication orders/prescriptions)
tot. prot.	total protein (laboratory/chemistry)
tox.	toxic toxicity toxin
TP	testosterone proprionate thrombocytopenic purpura thrombophlebitis total protein (laboratory/chemistry) Treponema pallidum (syphilis)
TPBF	total pulmonary blood flow

T^{Pe}	expiratory pause time (pulmonary function test)
T^{Pi}	inspiratory pause time (pulmonary function test)
TPI	Treponema pallidum-immobilization (test) (laboratory/serology)
TPIA	Treponema pallidum immune adherence (test) (laboratory/serology)
TPN	total parenteral nutrition (intravenous therapy)
TP & P	time, place, and person
TPR	temperature, pulse, respirations (vital signs) total peripheral resistance total pulmonary resistance
TPT	typhoid-paratyphoid (vaccine)
T(R)	temperature, rectal (on temperature records)
tr.	tincture (prescriptions) trace
trach.	tracheostomy
trach. asp.	tracheal aspiration
tract.	traction
train.	training
trans.	transverse
trans. d.	transverse diameter
transm.	transmission
transpı.	transplant (transplantation)

trans. sect.	transverse section
TRBF	total renal blood flow (renal function test)
Trep.	Treponema (on laboratory reports)
TRF	thyrotrophin releasing factor
TRH	thyrotrophin releasing hormone
TRIC	trachoma inclusive conjunctivitis
trig.	triglycerides (laboratory/chemistry)
tRNA	transfer ribonucleic acid
TRP	tubular reabsorption of phosphate (renal function test)
trt.	treatment
T$_3$RU	triiodothyronine resin uptake (laboratory/endocrinology)
TS	thoracic surgery tricuspid stenosis (heart)
TSD	Tay-Sachs disease
T-sect.	transverse (cross) section
T-set	tracheotomy set
TSH	thyroid stimulating hormone (laboratory/endocrinology)
TSH-RH	thyroid stimulating hormone-releasing factor (laboratory/endocrinology)
TSP	total serum protein
tsp.	teaspoon
T$_3$ SU	triiodothyronine serum uptake (laboratory/endocrinology)

TT	tetanus toxoid
	thrombin time
	thymol turbidity
	transthoracic
TTP	thrombotic thrombocytopenia purpura
TTT	tolbutamide tolerance test
tuberc.	tuberculosis
TUG	total urinary gonadotropin (laboratory/endocrinology)
T_3 uptake	triiodothyronine uptake (laboratory/endocrinology)
T_4 uptake	thyroxine uptake (laboratory/endocrinology)
TUR	transurethral resection (operation/urology)
TURP	transurethral resection of prostate (operation/urology)
tuss.	cough (Latin *tussis*)
TV	tidal volume (pulmonary function test)
	Trichomonas vaginalis (on bacteriology reports)
TVC	timed vital capacity (pulmonary function test)
	total volume capacity (pulmonary function test)
	triple voiding cystogram (procedure/urology)
TVH	total vaginal hysterectomy (operation/gynecology)
TVU	total volume urine

TW	tap water
Tx.	therapy traction (orthopedics) transfusion treatment
T & X	type and crossmatch (laboratory/blood bank)
tymp.	tympany
tymp. memb.	tympanic membrane
typ.	typical

U

U	unit (on laboratory reports) upper urology
u	units (on laboratory reports)
UA	uric acid (laboratory/chemistry) urine analysis (laboratory/urine)
UC	ulcerative colitis unit clerk urea clearance (renal function test) urethral catheter
U & C	urethral and cervical usual and customary
UCG	urinary chorionic gonadotropin (laboratory/endocrinology)
UCHD	usual childhood diseases
UCI	urethral catheter in

UCO	urethral catheter out
UD	unit dose urethral discharge
UE	upper extremity
UFA	unesterified (free) fatty acids (laboratory/chemistry)
UG	urogenital
UGI	upper gastrointestinal (series) (x-ray/esophagus, stomach, and duodenum)
UHF	ultrahigh frequency
UIBC	unsaturated iron-binding capacity (laboratory/chemistry)
UIQ	upper inner quadrant
UK	urokinase
UL	upper lobe
U & L	upper and lower
ult.	ultimate (ultimately)
UM	upper motor (neuron)
umb.	umbilicus (umbilical)
uncomp.	uncomplicated
uncon.	unconscious
uncond.	unconditioned
uncond. ref.	unconditioned reflex
uncorr.	uncorrected
undet. orig.	undetermined origin
ung.	ointment (Latin: *unguentum*) (prescriptions)
unilat.	unilateral

univ.	universal
unk.	unknown
unoff.	unofficial
unsat.	unsatisfactory
	unsaturated
UOQ	upper outer quadrant
UP	ureteropelvic
	uroporphyrin
U/P	urine-plasma ratio
up ad lib	out of bed, as desired
UPI	uteroplacental insufficiency
UPJ	ureteropelvic junction
UQ	upper quadrant
UR	unconditioned response
	upper respiratory
	utilization review
ur.	urine
URD	upper respiratory disease
ureth.	urethra (urethral)
URI	upper respiratory infection
uro-gen.	urogenital
Urol.	urology
URQ	upper right quadrant
URT	upper respiratory tract
URTI	upper respiratory tract infection
US	ultrasonic
USN	ultrasonic nebulizer (respiratory therapy)
U.S.P.	United States Pharmacopeia

UT	urinary tract
UTI	urinary tract infection
UU	urine urobilinogen (laboratory/chemistry)
UV	ultraviolet
	umbilical vein
	urine volume

V

V	vein
	Vibrio (on bacteriology reports)
	virus
	vision
	voice
	volume
	volume of gas (pulmonary function tests)
$\dot{V}$	rate of gas flow
	volume of gas per a unit of time (pulmonary function test)
v	volt
V1, V2, . . .	chest lead 1, chest lead 2, . . . (ECG)
VA	vacuum aspiration
	ventricular aneurysm
	vertebral artery
	Veterans Administration
	visual acuity (eye examination)
V_A	volume of alveolar gas (pulmonary function test)
$\dot{V}_A$	alveolar ventilation (pulmonary function test)
vac.	vacuum

vacc.	vaccinate (vaccination)
vag.	vagina (vaginal)
vag. hyst.	vaginal hysterectomy (operation/gynecology)
VAH	Veterans Administration Hospital
VAMP	vincristine, amethopterin, 6-mercaptopurine, and prednisone (cancer chemotherapy)
var.	variable variety various
vasc.	vascular
vas. dis.	vascular disease
VAT	ventricular activation time
VB	vertebral-basilar (arteries) viable birth
VBI	vertebral-basilar insufficiency
VBL	vinblastine (cancer chemotherapy)
VC	color vision (eye examination) vena cava ventilatory capacity (pulmonary function test) vital capacity (pulmonary function test) vocal cord
VCG	vectorcardiogram (procedure/cardiology)
VCR	vincristine (cancer chemotherapy)
VCT	venous clotting time (laboratory/coagulation)

VCU	voiding cystourethrogram (procedure/urology)
VD	venereal disease
V_D	volume of dead space gas (pulmonary function test)
VDA	visual discriminatory acuity
VdB test	Van den Bergh test (laboratory/chemistry)
VDG	venereal disease, gonorrhea
VDP	vincristine, daunorubicin, prednisone (cancer chemotherapy)
VDRL	Venereal Disease Research Laboratory (test for syphilis)
VDS	venereal disease, syphilis
VD/VT	ratio of dead space ventilation to total ventilation (pulmonary function test)
V_E	volume of expired gas (pulmonary function test)
$\dot{V}_E$	minute volume (pulmonary function test)
V & E	vinethene and ether (anesthetic agents)
VEB	ventricular ectopic beat (electrocardiogram)
vent.	ventilation ventricle (ventricular)
vent. fib.	ventricular fibrillation
ventr.	ventral
ventric.	ventricular

vert.	vertical
ves.	vessel
vesic.	vesicular
vest.	vestibular
VF	ventricular fibrillation
	visual field (eye examination)
	vocal fremitus
VG	ventricular gallop (rhythm)
V/G	very good
VGM	ventriculogram (procedure/cardiology)
VH	vaginal hysterectomy (operation/gynecology)
	viral hepatitis
VHD	valvular heart disease
VHF	visual half-field (eye examination)
vib.	vibration
VIP	very important person
vis.	vision (visual)
	visitor
visc.	visceral
	viscosity
	viscous
Vit.	vitamin
vit.	vital
vit. cap.	vital capacity (pulmonary function test)
viz	namely (Latin: *videlicet*)
VJ	ventriculojugular (shunt)
VM	vestibular membrane

VMA	vanillylmandelic acid (laboratory/endocrinology)
V/O	verbal order
VOD	vision right eye (eye examination)
vol.	volume voluntary
VOS	vision left eye (eye examination)
VP	venous pressure
VPB	ventricular premature beat
VPC	ventricular premature contraction
VPRC	volume of packed red cells (laboratory/hematology)
v.p.s.	vibrations per second
V/Q	ventilation-perfusion ratio (pulmonary function test)
VR	ventricular rate
VRI	viral respiratory infection
VS	venesection vesicular sounds
V/S	vital signs
vs.	versus
VSD	ventricular septal defect (heart)
VSS	vital signs stable
VT	ventricular tachycardia
V_T	tidal volume (pulmonary function test) total ventilation (pulmonary function test)
V & V	vulva and vagina
v/v	volume for volume

VWD	von Willebrand's disease
vx.	vertex
VZ	varicella-zoster

W

W	white
	widow
	widower
	width
	wife
Wass.	Wassermann test (for syphilis) (laboratory/serology)
WB	Wechsler-Bellevue Scale (psychological test)
	weight bearing
	whole blood
	whole body
WBC	white blood count (laboratory/hematology)
WBC/hpf	white blood cells per high power field (on urinalysis reports)
WBPTT	whole blood partial thromboplastin time
WC	ward clerk
	wheel chair
	white count (laboratory/hematology)
WD	well developed
	well differentiated
	wet dressing
Wd.	ward

WDHA	watery diarrhea with hypokalemia and achlorhydria
wds.	wounds
WD/WN	well developed, well nourished
WEE	Western equine encephalitis
WF	white female
wh.	white
whpl.	whirlpool (procedure/physical therapy)
wid.	widow (widower)
WK	Wernicke-Korsakoff (syndrome)
wk.	weak week
WL	waiting list
WL test	waterload test (procedure/endocrinology)
WM	white male
WN	well nourished
WNF	well nourished female
WNL	within normal limits
WNM	well nourished male
W/O	written order
w/o	without
WPW	Wolff-Parkinson-White (syndrome)
wr.	wrist
w/s	watt-seconds
wt.	weight
w/u	work-up

WV	whispered voice
w/v	weight per volume

X

X	cross or transverse magnification times
x	axis (of cylindrical lens)
x3, x4, . . .	3 times, 4 times, . . .
x2d, x3d, . . .	for 2 days, for 3 days, . . . (medication orders/prescriptions)
xanth.	xanthomatosis
X factor	an unidentified factor
X-match	cross-match (laboratory/blood bank)
XT	exotropic (eye examination)
XX chromosome	normal female chromosome type
XY chromosome	normal male chromosome type
Xyl.	xylose

Y

yel.	yellow
YO	years old
YOB	year of birth
yr.	year
YS	yellow spot (of the retina)

Z

Z	zero
ZE syndrome	Zollinger-Ellison syndrome
ZIG	zoster immune globulin

SYMBOLS

+ or ⊕	plus positive present
?	possible questionable question of
− or ⊖	absent minus negative
↑	up
↑	above elevated greater than increase (increases) rising
↓	below decrease (decreases) falling less than
>	greater than
<	less than
≤	less than or equal to
≥	greater than or equal to
≅	approximately

∼	approximate
=	equals
Δ	change
±	either positive or negative plus or minus very slight trace
+	slight trace (or reaction)
+ +	trace (or noticeable reaction)
+ + +	moderate amount (or reaction)
+ + + +	large amount (or pronounced reaction)
+ reaction	acid reaction
− reaction	alkaline reaction
→	results in (is due to) to the right transfer to
←	to the left
↑↑	extensor response, Babinski sign (neurological examination)
↓↓	plantar response, Babinski sign (neurological examination)
↓↓	testes descended
↑↑	testes undescended
$\widehat{m}$	murmur
℞	prescription take
ʒ	dram (teaspoonful) (medication orders/prescriptions)
$f\,ʒ$	fluid dram (medication orders/prescriptions)

℥	ounce (medication order)
f℥	fluid ounce (medication orders/prescriptions)
ϯ	one
ϯϯ	two
1x	once
2x	twice
°	degree
1°	first degree primary
2°	secondary second degree
2ndry	secondary
'	foot minute
"	inch second
Δt	time interval
24°	24 hours
$\sqrt{}$	square root
$\sqrt[3]{}$	cube root
$\sqrt{c}$	check with
#	number pound
@	at
.	ratio
::	proportionate to
/	per

♂	male
○○	male
♀	female
○	female
†	death
*	birth
⊙	start of operation (on anesthesia records)
X	start of anesthesia (on anesthesia records)
⊗	end of anesthesia (on anesthesia records)
V	systolic blood pressure (on anesthesia records)
Λ	diastolic blood pressure (on anesthesia records)
○	respirations (on anesthesia records)
•	pulse rate (on anesthesia records)
Δ	temperature (on anesthesia records)
S	suction (on anesthesia records)
λ	wave length
μc	microcurie
μEq	microequivalent
μf	microfarad
μg	microgram (1/1000 of milligram)
μμg	micromicrogram (picogram)

$\mu\mu$	micromicron
μM	micromolar
μ	micron
μsec	microsecond
μv	microvolt
μw	microwatt
μV	milligamma
mμc	millimicrogram (nanocurie)
mμ	millimicron

Other Abbreviations